THE
Essential
CANNABIS
BOOK

Text © 2018 by Rob Mejia

Photographs © 2018 by photographers as listed on page 177

Publisher: Paul McGahren
Editorial Director: Matthew Teague
Editor: Kerri Grzybicki
Design: Lindsay Hess
Layout: Jodie Delohery

Spring House Press
P.O. Box 239
Whites Creek, TN 37189

ISBN: 978-1-940611-81-5

Library of Congress Control Number: 2018955135

Printed in The United States of America

10 9 8 7 6 5 4 3 2 1

Note: The following list contains names used in *The Essential Cannabis Book* that may be registered with the United States Copyright Office: University of Kansas, Bugatti Veyron, Jaguar, Bentley, BMW 3, BMW 5, Mercedes A Klasse, Mercedes C Klasse, Mercedes S Klasse, Oxycodone, Fentanyl, Adderall, Tylenol, Marinol, Xanax, Valium, Ambien, Ativan, Soma, Eli Lily, Parke-Davis, Brothers Smith, Tildens, Dupont, OxyContin, Frontline, AARP, CNN, ACLU, Human Rights Watch, G-7, Rastafarian, Malawi Gold, NAACP, Yale, Ameriprise Financial, Goldman Sachs, Project Equity, Columbia University, *Entrepreneur Magazine,* Forbes, Forbes 30 Under 30 List, Full Color 50, The Hood Incubator, EARTH Law LLC, Google, Marquette University, NORML, Oregon State University, Lewis and Clark Law School, Hemp History Week, *Fordham Environmental Law Review,* Relegalizing Industrial Hemp Project, Volkswagen, Volkswagen Bug, *Fast Times at Ridgemont High,* Cheech and Chong, Motrin, Pure Hemp Collective, *DOPE Magazine,* Defending Our Patients Everywhere, Hempfest, Afghani, Durban Poison, Sour Diesel, Blue Dream, Super Silver Haze, Purple Haze, OG Sour Diesel, Maui Waui, Granddaddy Purple, Northern Lights, Master Kush, Purple Urkel, G-13, Hindu Kush, Hashplant, Chronic, White Widow, AK-47, Blueberry, Purple Kush, Pineapple Express, Strawberry Cough, Bubble Gum, Juicy Fruit, Purple Skunk, Ringo's Gift, ACDC, Harle-Tsu, Stephen Hawking Kush, Cannatonic, Harlequin, Canna-Tsu, Pennywise, Sour Tsunami, Sweet and Sour Widow, Stanley Brothers, Charlotte's Web, Anheuser-Busch, Marinol, Sativex, GW Pharmaceuticals, Americans for Safe Access, ASA, University of Mississippi, University of Arizona, Cannabis Grand Cru, University of Virginia Law School, Kindle, Denver Post, University of Connecticut, *Journal of Addiction, British Journal of Clinical Pharmacology, Entourage,* Harold and Kumar, Point Seven Group, D.A.R.E, Back Door Medicine, Girl Scout, *Reefer Madness,* Stashlogix, CanopyBoulder, Our Community Harvest, The Cannabist, tCheck2, Nova, Levo, MagicalButter, MB2e, Herb, *The Ganja Kitchen Revolution, Wake and Bake, Dazed and Infused,* Kalamata, Tabasco, Nellie & Joe's, Grateful Dead, Aspen Police Department, Splinter, VETCBD, Federal Deposit Insurance Corporation, Cannabis Now, Future Cannabis Project, Laurie and Mary Jane, Leafly, Marijuana Policy Project, National Hemp Association, NORML, Project CBD, Beatles, *Paul McCartney: Many Years to Come, Sanford & Son, Three's Company, Different Strokes.*

The author and publisher believe the facts in the book are accurate as of the date of production. However, the content of the book could include technical inaccuracies or other errors.

The information and opinions found here are based on the author's experiences, research, and anecdotal information. This book is not intended to provide legal advice or guidance. The use and distribution of cannabis is governed by laws that vary widely, and these actions remain illegal in many places. Readers are responsible for consulting their own professional legal advice about the current state of the laws applicable to their own location and circumstances.

This book is not intended to provide medical or health advice, diagnosis, or treatment. Nor is this book intended to cover all possible uses, precautions, directions, or adverse effects involving cannabis. Statements and claims about possible health benefits or effects discussed in this book have not been evaluated by the U.S. Food and Drug Administration. Readers should not disregard or postpone seeking professional advice relating to any condition because of statements found in this book. Readers are responsible for consulting their own health care professionals before following any ideas in this book.

Readers are advised that the use of products and information discussed in the book is done solely at their own risk. The author and the publisher do not assume, and specifically disclaim, any responsibility for any loss, damage, injury, or other consequences resulting from any reader's use or application of any of the information discussed in the book.

To learn more about Spring House Press books, or to find a retailer near you, email info@springhousepress.com or visit us at www.springhousepress.com.

THE
Essential
CANNABIS
BOOK

ROB MEJIA

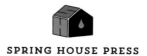

SPRING HOUSE PRESS

DEDICATION

To Beth Ann, with love

ACKNOWLEDGMENTS

So many people contributed to this book in ways great and small. The best parts of the book are theirs and I can never express my appreciation for all the love and support I've received.
In particular, I'd like to thank:

My six amazing sons, Chris, Grant, Nick, Myles, Maxx, and Dante.

My parents, David and Ophelia, who made us all feel special though we grew up as an army of 13 kids!

My siblings and their families: Mary, Dave, Annie, Theresa (whose sad passing started me on my cannabis journey), Patty, Margaret, Pauline, James, Louise, Shatta, Catherine, and Tom.

The members and contributors to Our Community Harvest LLC, namely Andrea, our CBD expert; Robert, who was there in an advisory capacity every step of the way; and especially Dan, who drove every OCH project with zeal, intelligence, and creativity; his imprint is all over these pages.

Irv Rosenfeld, who graciously wrote the foreword, contributed a sidebar, and was patient as I peppered him with question after question.

Home cannacook Corinne Tobias, who contributed infusing knowledge, recipes, and a bunch of good humor. Her helpful, entertaining Web site is www.wakeandbake.co.

In addition to Irv and Corinne, the sidebar contributors, listed below, put a human face and story on all things cannabis. Their stories are personal, important, and inspiring. I admire their courage and grit:

Aspen Sheriff Joe DiSalvo; *Dope Magazine* co-founder, James Zachodni; Juliet Fillweber and Terri Leek, mothers and owners of Pure Hemp Collective; Mitch Meyers, a dispensary owner and CBD provider in Missouri; Anthony Dittmann (and Hez Blake), co-founders of Cannabis Grand Cru, an educational cannabis events company; Dr. Barney Warf, University of Kansas geography professor; Sister Kate, grower, CBD producer, healer, and head of the compassionate cannabis organization, Sisters of the Valley; Andrea Dow, CBD educator and patient; Courtney Moran, hemp attorney; Paula-Noel Macfie, Ph.D., researcher and founder of Back Door Medicine, specializing in the use of suppositories; Ashley Picillo, author of *Breaking the Grass Ceiling* (a collection of 21 profiles of women in cannabis) and founder and CEO of Point Seven Group; Robert Martinez, New Mexico medical patient and accomplished home grower; Dr. Tim Shu, veterinarian and owner of PETCBD; Skip Stone, co-founder of Stashlogix, products to keep cannabis safely stored from kids and pets; Ebele Ifedigbo, co-creator of The Hood Incubator, who

> *"I may not have gone where I intended to go, but I think I have ended up where I intended to be."*
>
> —Douglas Adams

helps people of color get a foothold in the cannabis business; Shatta Mejia, home cannacook and supportive brother; and Jessie Gill, the holistic nurse known as Marijuana Mommy.

Other individuals who were gracious with their time and expertise include:

Chef Laurie, Mary, and Bruce, who welcomed me into their home and who taught me how to cook with cannabis and to appreciate cannabis photography. Scott, Wanda, and Randy, who lent so much of their time and cooking/advocacy expertise as I was getting started in the industry. Ricardo, who has encyclopedic knowledge about cannabis and is one of the best journalists I know. Renae L., whose curiosity makes her a great cannabis conversationalist and also happens to be a master hair stylist. Bob, who has a strong understanding of state regulations regarding CBD and who answered many of my first questions.

My anchors and friends: Chris and Meg, Mike and Emily, Brad and Karen, Brian, Chris and Stacy, Jeff and Heather, Gwen, Theresa and Bill, Peter and Traci, John and Pam, Patrick and Laura, John S. and Laura, Jim M., Lee L., Jessie and Susie, Tina, Michaela H., John G. and Suzanne, Matt and Jill P., John and Andrea C., John R., Rob F., Tim R., Annie, Jane M., Shannon, Marie G., Carrie B., Vanessa, Larry H. (who gave me a consulting job just when I needed it), Ted W., Jon K., and Kate M.

My friends in the licensing business: Michael and Lindsay, James, Phil, Karen, Kim, Liz, Michael C., Greg and Bob, Nicholas and Linda, David B., Elise, Michael S., Juan, Darren, Jeff, and Andrew.

My tennis friends and students, who literally keep me on my toes, and show great patience and insight when we talk about cannabis: Rob, Dr. Jeff A., Bob B., Jeff B., Kyle and Emilie, Alex, Peter C., Jo and Carol, Bruce, Tom F., Hy, Tom H., John C. H., Bill H., Kenny K., Bob and JoAnn K., Mark L., Holly M., Paul, Kim and Linda, Tom M., David M., Scott, Greg, Beth and Peter, Dianne N., Roberto, Sean, Ray P., Doug, Mike P., Billy P., Ronnie, Richie S., Modeste, Peter S. (whose expertise and opinions were timely), Bonnie W., Peter and Bridget, Richie W., Dave W., Duncan, my doubles partner Alan, Bob G., Norm, Dr. John C., and of course, my tennis students at Quest, whose lessons are equal parts laughter and technique.

The remarkable staff at Spring House Press, who believed in this project from the beginning. It is such a pleasure to work with a publisher who supports, nurtures, and shares an author's vision. My sincere thanks go to: Paul, Matthew, Kerri, Lindsay, and Jodie.

"This is U.S. History; I see the globe right there."
—Jeff Spicoli

FOREWORD

This book is a fantastic guide to help you learn about the medical benefits of cannabis and how it can apply to everyone's life. I have read many books on this subject and this one is the most down-to-earth.

I personally discovered the medical benefits of cannabis quite by accident in the fall of 1971. I wish there had been a book like this one available to have helped me with my struggles taking on Uncle Sam. I helped pioneer this movement so books like this one could be written to help educate more people.

Rob has touched on most of the amazing aspects of this plant and how it can be ingested. So many people think that it has to be lit up and smoked to be effective. He explains other ways of taking this medicine and why it still works.

So many books have been written by so-called experts in this field and all of them make some good points. However, so many writers make it very difficult to understand because they are experts. This book is written by people who are "living experts": people who have lived and experienced it, not simply studied it.

Everyone who has made a difference in this worldwide movement has their own story to tell. I hope this book will pique your interest to read more about this unique plant and the people who have gotten us to where we are today.

Cannabis is still a Schedule I drug in the U.S. as of 2018, with no accepted medical use. While today it is available in many states, patients are still being arrested for the use of a substance that the federal government has been giving me since 1982.

We need more people to learn about this remarkable medicine and help educate more people so one day, all patients nationwide will have the same rights and easy access that I have.

Learn from what Rob has put in the following pages. Realize you *can* make a difference on this important issue.

It has been an honor to introduce this book to you. Thank you for your interest. Spread the word to all: Cannabis works!

— *Irvin Rosenfeld*

The longest surviving of the final two federal medical cannabis patients in the U.S. (read more on page 70).

An Open Letter to Moms, Dads, Guardians, Friends, Etc. (of Cannabis Users)

Dear Loved Ones:

Your sons, daughters, nieces, nephews, uncles, aunts, grandparents, and friendly neighbors are smoking, eating, drinking, infusing their food, and using topical cannabis. Or they are very curious about doing so. But before you get too upset, it is my hope that you'll read this book, gain a little knowledge, and begin an informed conversation. I'm looking forward to it.

Did you know that:

* Cannabis was legal in the U.S. until 1937
* 43% of all U.S. adults have tried cannabis (Gallup, Inc. 2016)
* Among adult users, 54% are parents (Marist Poll 2017)
* 80% of older adults support use of medical cannabis with a doctor's consent (Gabriel 2018)
* Sales of CBD products have increased at a rate of 100% per year from 2014 to 2017 and show no signs of slowing (BDS Analytics 2017)
* Cannabis may have been one of the first plants that humans domesticated/farmed
* Cannabis grows naturally in most parts of the world that are not too cold

It is only legal to grow hemp in about two-thirds of the U.S. (plus a few states have started test or pilot programs), but we import a great deal of hemp and hemp seeds from China, Canada, Latin American countries like Chile and Uruguay, and France.

As we learn more and more about this intriguing plant, you may want to consider how it could benefit you. If you have stress (ha! show me someone who has no stress), or perhaps your knees ache, or you have trouble sleeping, or you experience anxiety, you may be a good candidate for cannabis. There are ways to experience the benefits of cannabis, even if you don't want to get high. And, it is natural.

But whatever you think of cannabis now, if I've done my job, by the time you finish reading this book, you will learn a few things about this magnificent plant and will understand—or at least become curious about—its booming popularity.

Much love,
Your Cannabis Sons, Daughters, Nieces, Nephews, Uncles, Aunts, Grandparents, and Friendly Neighbors

P.S. Mom, last time we talked you said you like surprises. How did I do?

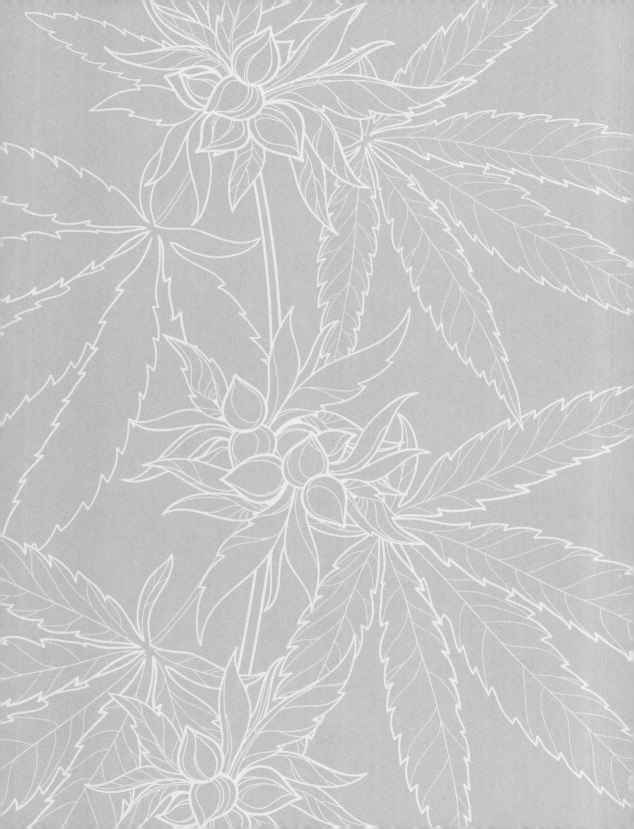

CONTENTS

INTRODUCTION

If you had asked me several years ago what type of book I would be most likely to write, it would not have been a general introduction to cannabis. But then my world was shaken when my older sister Theresa got cancer. As her body deteriorated, she was put on more and more meds until she didn't know where or who she was. When family members visited in her final days, we talked a lot about care options and the use of medical cannabis came up again and again. The topic may have come up because a large part of my family still lives in Colorado—home of the first state to legalize recreational cannabis back in 2012. It was at that time my brothers and I began to not only see but start to explore the great possibilities and potential in cannabis. It was at that time I started my journey into the cannabis community.

Cannabis legalization, whether medical or recreational, is growing, as is the research. In this emerging environment, reports on the medical possibilities of cannabis, especially as a natural alternative to traditional pain treatments, are increasing. Not only states but entire countries—hello Uruguay and Canada!—are legalizing and embracing recreational cannabis. Recently, Vermont became the first state to legalize cannabis via the legislature instead of popular vote; New Jersey and New Hampshire are expected to follow shortly. States are opening up hemp production for the first time in decades. Chefs are specializing in cooking with cannabis. There are even a number of studies saying that a compound found in cannabis, CBD (cannabidiol, pronounced can-na-bid-e-all) can be used to treat inflammation, anxiety, and other common conditions without getting the user high. And unlike recreational marijuana, CBD is legal across the U.S. and is available in many forms. Any way you look at it, there is a lot going on.

Like you, I am curious. And thanks to a globally connected world, I have been able to feed my curiosity by speaking with an amazing community of people. My journey has been filled with remarkable characters, great stories, and incredible experiences. I have been able to apprentice with an accomplished cannabis chef in Oregon and experience a cannabis club in Uruguay. I have spoken with CBD-growing nuns in California, a pro-cannabis sheriff in Colorado, and

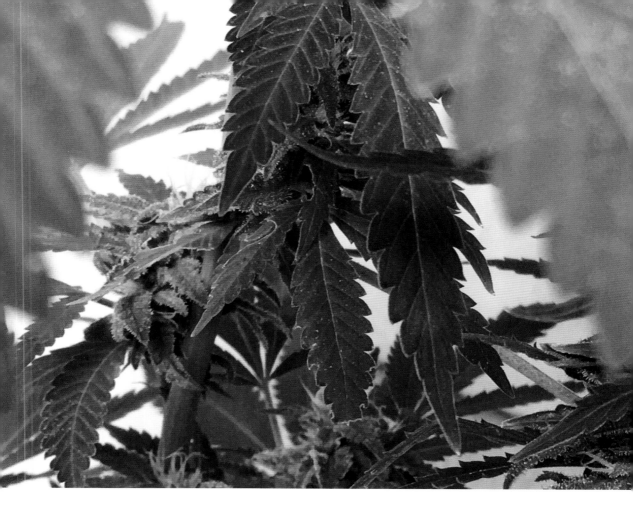

a hemp attorney in Portland. I have met people for whom cannabis is a godsend—relieving pain, controlling seizures, mitigating tumors, and stimulating appetite where other treatments couldn't. But what surprised me the most was how many people around me shared my curiosity. From the guys I play tennis with to my friends with parents suffering from joint pain, my questions were their questions. This book is the offspring of my journey and our questions.

Whether you are interested in recreational or medical use, getting high or not getting high, cooking with cannabis, or simply becoming more educated, my goal is to provide enough knowledge for you to be comfortable in this new pro-cannabis world and to give you the strategies to continue to learn.

—Rob Mejia

Chapter 1
THE HISTORY OF CANNABIS

Cannabis is one of the most successful plants around. Like many plants used for nourishment, pain relief, and pleasure for eons, cannabis grows wild in many parts of the world. And it is big, big business. It is estimated that the legal market for cannabis in 2020 in the U.S. will surpass 44 billion dollars! These numbers are largely driven by adult recreational (and to a lesser degree, medical) users and grew by 26% over the previous year. In 2017, Colorado, which was the first state to legalize recreational cannabis, exceeded 1.5 billion dollars in legal sales and gained about 300 million dollars in tax revenue.

Other nations that grow an impressive amount of cannabis include Colombia and Mexico (which export a sizable percentage of their crops to the U.S.), India (but not much product is exported), Afghanistan (the single largest producer in the world), South Africa, the Netherlands, and Kazakhstan. Recent figures also show the UK has become a major medical cannabis producer. This is surprising, as the UK does not allow for recreational nor medical use. But as mentioned, cannabis is a diverse plant that grows wild in many different climates. I have witnessed this first hand; I have a friend in Costa Rica, and on his tree farm there are three cannabis plants (that he never planted) that are healthy, resiny, and well over 12 feet tall! I should make plans to visit him again soon.

Cannabis has been around in the wild for centuries and was reportedly cultivated in China as early as 500 B.C. Many cultures, including the Rastafarians of Jamaica and the Hindus of India (who drink a special buttermilk-like cannabis drink, byang) have developed deep relationships with this plant over an extended period of time. Today, most cannabis cultivation is large-scale production mostly relegated to the indoors, where smart, passionate growers are continually improving upon and creating new strains, each designed for specific experiences.

On a personal note, of everyone I met during my journey, the growers were probably the most learned, creative, sometimes slightly crazy members of the cannabis community. I am in awe of what they know and can do. They have honed their craft so well they can get the plant to bloom and bear fruit earlier, in remarkable quantities, and often with greater potency. But they are not just helping plants to grow healthier and stronger. Many growers and their elected representatives are also at the forefront of pushing on antiquated policies, such as banking laws and the discrepancies between state and federal legislation, to move the industry forward. Colorado House Representative Ed Perlmutter introduced a bill, twice, that proposed legitimate banking services for cannabis industries that run a legal, state-regulated business. But so far, the Rules Committee has blocked the legislation from even coming up for a vote. Perlmutter has now banded with Congressional Representatives from Alaska and Washington, and continues to push fair banking legislation for the cannabis industry (Permutter 2017).

Although the U.S. is a relatively new nation, cannabis has been around from the beginning. We have a complicated history with marijuana, filled with love, then hate, then love again. But clearly the cannabis story didn't start with the birth of our nation.

Older History of Cannabis

The story of cannabis starts in China. The first reference to marijuana comes from China, where in 2737 B.C. Emperor Shen Nung mentions its promise as medicine; he writes that it aids gout, rheumatism, constipation, and other medical conditions (Joy and Mack 2001, 9).

Ramses II and his contemporaries were apparently aware of the medici-nal value of cannabis as well, because cannabis pollen dated 1213 B.C. was found on the entombed body of Ramses II. The Egyptians were ahead of their time because their uses for cannabis included the treatment of glaucoma, administering enemas, cooling the uterus, and controlling inflammation (Manniche 1989).

Cannabis was apparently introduced to Europe by the Scythians (who came from present day Kazakhstan) around A.D. 500; a pot containing seeds and leaves was found near Berlin. Around that time, cannabis circulated all throughout Northern Europe.

According to Martin Booth in his illustrative book titled *Cannabis: A History:* "During the Middle Ages, hemp was central to any herbalist's medicine cabinet. William Turner, the naturalist considered the first English botanist, praises it in his *New Herball,* published in 1538." Turner wrote simply that cannabis was a healing herb.

Cannabis moved around the world from cultures who embraced the plant to new arrivals who saw its potential. For example, when Napoleon invaded Egypt in 1799, he brought along a group of scientists who discovered the Rosetta Stone. Guess what else they did? They took cannabis back home with them. Their investigation and study

Profile

THE RACIST ROOTS OF CANNABIS PROHIBITION

DR. BARNEY WARF, *University of Kansas, Geography Department*

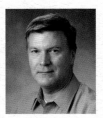

I am a professor and have spent my career in academia. I am also a scholar of cannabis and an outspoken advocate for its legalization. I came to view cannabis not simply in personal terms, but as a social issue deeply intertwined with debates over social justice, inequality, racial relations, and imprisonment.

As an adolescent, I smoked cannabis simply because it was fun. Yet, as a social scientist, I gradually came to see cannabis as something more than a source of pleasure. I became curious about its history, how it entered the U.S., and why it was illegal. It dawned on me that the war against cannabis was about something greater; that is, about racial injustice and the dysfunctional American judicial system. From the beginning, attempts to criminalize it were based on racist stereotypes. The war on cannabis is largely a war on racial minorities. Caring about this injustice led me to advocate cannabis legalization as a human rights issue. The federal government subsidized tobacco for years, which has killed millions, yet classifies cannabis as a Schedule I drug, along with heroin and LSD, although there has never been a confirmed case of anyone dying from using it. The hypocrisy and denial of science, let alone the horrific impacts on people's lives, are intolerable.

To view cannabis in this light—in social terms—is to shed light on the racist politics that underpin the war against it.

The Geographic Flow of Cannabis Around the World, courtesy Dr. Barney Warf.

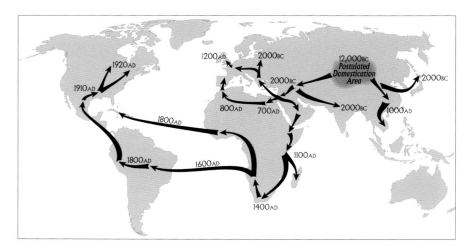

of cannabis led them to discover its pain-relieving and sedative properties. This was just one more step towards the acceptance of cannabis in Western medicine (National Commission on Marihuana and Drug Abuse 1972).

The History of Cannabis in the United States

In the U.S., cannabis has an equally fascinating history. The Spanish brought marijuana to the U.S. around 1545. Hemp, a sturdy plant that was easy to grow and extremely versatile, quickly became a popular crop (Booth 2005). It was more than popular; it was required. The Jamestown colonists were ordered by the British to grow hemp in 1619; each landowner had to cultivate 100 hemp plants for

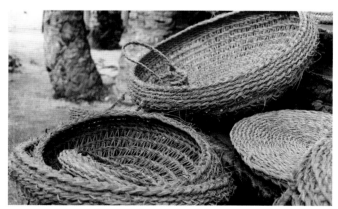

Hemp can do it all. Hemp fabric is more durable than cotton and can be used in clothes and textiles of all type. It can also be woven into strong ropes and cables that are capable of very heavy lifting and pulling.

export. A decade later, Massachusetts and Connecticut landowners were required to grow hemp as well.

Hemp is woven into the fabric of America, literally and figuratively. From colonial times to the 1800s, it was estimated that well over 70% of U.S. woven goods were made from hemp. A surprising number of products can be made from hemp, including building materials, industrial lubricants, paper, health and beauty aids, and all types of ropes and fabrics. In fact, if you drive a Bugatti Veyron, Jaguar, Bentley, BMW 3 or 5, or Mercedes A, C, or S Klasse, your driver's side panel door is constructed of hemp fiber, which is a strong and lightweight material. More about hemp is covered later in the chapter.

Another milestone for cannabis is its listing in the prestigious publication *U.S. Pharmacopoeia,* a book whose goal was to standardize the uses of botanicals in medicine (Booth 2005, 659). From 1850 to 1937, marijuana was recognized as a remedy for numerous ailments. According to Richard Glen Boire, JD and Kevin Feeney, JD in their publication *Medical Marijuana Law:* "By 1850, marijuana had made its way into the *U.S. Pharmacopeia* [an official public standards-setting authority for all prescription and over-the-counter medicines], which listed marijuana as treatment for numerous afflictions, including: neuralgia, tetanus, typhus, cholera, rabies, dysentery, alcoholism, opiate addiction, anthrax, leprosy, incontinence, gout, convulsive disorders, tonsillitis, insanity, excessive menstrual bleeding, and uterine bleeding, among others."

It is interesting to note that opioid addiction was listed as a condition that could benefit from cannabis because today there is a vigorous debate as to whether cannabis is a good and viable replacement for opioids; there is also evidence that some opioid users do benefit from cannabis use.

This means that from 1850 to roughly 1937, medical cannabis was available in many forms. It was produced by large pharmaceutical companies like Eli Lilly, Parke-Davis, Brothers Smith, and Tildens. At that point, one of the most popular products were tinctures (or drops). Interestingly, this form of medical cannabis is wildly popular today, especially for people who would prefer not to smoke. Not surprisingly, after the Marijuana Act of 1937 effectively stopped production and marked the beginning of the villainization of cannabis, it was made even more official when cannabis was then removed from the *U.S. Pharmacopeia* in 1942.

As mentioned, the Marijuana Tax Act of 1937 nearly dealt recreation-

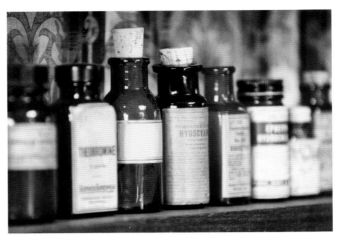

History repeats itself. In the last half of the 19th and early part of the 20th century, medicinal marijuana was widely prescribed. As laws change and preconceptions are disproved, the same thing is beginning to happen.

al and medical cannabis and hemp a death blow, effectively stopping production by putting penalties in place for both users and growers. And like so many ill-advised policies, this one started with cultural misunderstanding and racism. Beginning in 1910, there was a huge influx of Mexican immigrants looking for work or fleeing political violence during and after the Mexican Revolution. They used marijuana after a day's work for medicine and relaxation. And even though cannabis was present in many American medicines at the time, "marijuana"—a new, foreign, dangerous word and product—alarmed many and an active campaign to ban marihuana/marijuana began. These attitudes were exacerbated by a "jazz culture" in many urban cities where musicians were known to partake as well. Propaganda, in the form of sensationalistic movies such as *Reefer Madness*, fueled the fire of mistrust. There are also suggestions that Dupont lobbied for a ban on marijuana in order to cripple the hemp trade. As the story goes, Dupont had developed synthetic fibers, including nylon, and the ban was one opportunistic way to gain market share.

In 1970, Congress, acting under then-President Richard Nixon passed the Controlled Substances Act (CSA) as a component of the Comprehensive Drug Abuse Prevention and Control Act. Five schedules were created, and cannabis was vengefully placed in a list of Schedule I drugs along with heroin and LSD. Schedule I drugs have "no currently accepted medical use" and have a high potential for abuse. Even methadone, cocaine, and OxyContin are not listed as Schedule I drugs, but as Schedule II drugs (DEA, "Drug Scheduling").

Schedule I: Drugs with no currently accepted medical use and a high potential for abuse. They are the most dangerous drugs of all the drug schedules with potentially severe psychological or physical dependence.

Schedule II: Drugs with a high potential for abuse, with use potentially leading to severe psychological or physical dependence. These drugs are also considered dangerous.

Schedule III: Drugs with a moderate to low potential for physical and psychological dependence. Schedule III drugs' abuse potential is less than Schedule I and Schedule II drugs, but more than Schedule IV.

Schedule IV: Drugs with a low potential for abuse and low risk of dependence.

Schedule V: Drugs with lower potential for abuse than Schedule IV

Schedule I	Schedule II	Schedule III	Schedule IV	Schedule V
Marijuana	Cocaine	Tylenol (w/codeine)	Xanax	Robitussin
LSD	Methamphetamine	Ketamine	Valium	Lyrica
Heroin	Oxycodone	Anabolic steroids	Ambien	Parepectolin
Ecstasy	Fentanyl	Testosterone	Ativan	Motofen
Peyote	Adderall	Marinol (synthetic cannabis)	Soma	Lomotil

and consist of preparations containing limited quantities of certain narcotics. Schedule V drugs are generally used for antidiarrheal, antitussive, and analgesic purposes (DEA "A Tradition" and "Drug Scheduling").

In 1972, following on the heels of the creation of the CSA, Nixon commissioned a report on Marijuana and Drug Abuse known as the Shafer Commission. Former Republican Governor Raymond Shafer headed the committee, and after extensive study, the commission determined that the personal use of cannabis should be decriminalized, and penalties levied on non-violent drug offenders should be reviewed. This was not at all what Nixon expected; he was livid with the findings and simply ignored the report and its recommendations (Frontline 1998).

I'm sure many of you remember the ubiquitous 1980s anti-drug slogan "Just Say No" (to drugs) and the famous commercial of an egg frying in a pan with an ominous announcer saying, "this is your brain on drugs." This sentiment—which contributed to the demonization of cannabis—was furthered by the Comprehensive Crime Control Act of 1984 and the Anti-Drug Abuse Act of 1986. The Comprehensive Crime Control Act increased federal penalties for simple possession and dealing and the Anti-Drug Abuse Act instituted mandatory sentencing and a requirement that three offenses meant a life sentence for repeat drug offenders and the death penalty for "drug kingpins" (Frontline 1998).

Why are attitudes toward cannabis changing?

In the U.S., medical marijuana became legal for the first time in late 1996 in California via Proposition 215. Under this provision, if a California citizen obtained a physician's recommendation, the patient could possess and grow cannabis as long as they were receiving treatment for cancer, anorexia, AIDS, chronic pain, spasticity, glaucoma, arthritis, migraine, or any other illness for which cannabis was recommended by their doctor (Joy and Mack 2001).

Medical cannabis legalization in California was the beginning of a major shift in public attitudes, as shortly thereafter—in 1998—the states of Alaska, Oregon, and Washington legalized medical marijuana as well. To demonstrate this point more fully, an AARP poll in 2018 found that 80% of seniors support cannabis with a doctor's recommendation and 62% believe health insurance should cover medical cannabis. This poll also revealed that roughly 30% of respondents had tried cannabis at some point in their lives.

Profile

MY PERSONAL RELATIONSHIP WITH THE CANNABIS PLANT

SISTER KATE, *Sister of the Valley, Sellers of Cannabinoid Tinctures and Salves*

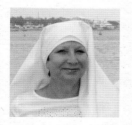

When I was only 40 years old, I started experiencing serious menopause symptoms. I had recently made a major change and moved my whole family across the ocean to Amsterdam. It was a big change with three children under age five and a budding consulting firm to run. The stress from it all threw me into premature menopause, the doctors mused. It was the sleeplessness that was making me crazy and I complained to my doctor that the sleeplessness was going to ruin my marriage. He asked me if I ever smoked cannabis and when I said I had, recreationally, he said I should try having it "medically" before going to bed—a whole joint. He also advised me to give up alcohol and caffeine, and it turned out to be a winning combination. I got my life back because I got my sleep back.

A decade later, I used the cannabis plant to get my nephew off of heroin. He had been using for more than five years when I got him.

I also moved to California and founded a Sisterhood that grows and makes healing products out of high-CBD cannabis. We believe the cannabis plant is most effective when combined with other health-taking measures. We believe the cannabis plant to be intelligent and cooperative. You can, for example, be putting any kind of pharmaceuticals into your body and the plant medicine cooperates with that; you can be trying to reverse cancer through diet and cannabis would cooperate with that.

Then, in a highly publicized TV event, Dr. Sanjay Gupta, who has become an outspoken proponent of the use of medical cannabis, apologized on CNN for his lack of support for medical cannabis. In his own words, "I mistakenly believed the Drug Enforcement Agency listed marijuana as a Schedule I substance because of sound scientific proof. Surely, they must have quality reasoning as to why marijuana is in the category of the most dangerous drugs that have 'no accepted medicinal use and a high potential for abuse.' They didn't have the science to support that claim, and I now know that when it comes to marijuana, neither of those things are true. It doesn't have a high potential for abuse, and there are very legitimate medical applications...We have been terribly and systematically misled for nearly 70 years in the United States, and I apologize for my own role in that" (Gupta 2013).

Thirty states plus the District of Columbia have medical cannabis programs: Alaska, Arizona, Arkansas, California, Colorado, Connecticut, Delaware, Florida, Hawaii, Illinois, Maine, Maryland, Massachusetts, Michigan, Minnesota, Montana, Nevada, New Hampshire, New Jersey, New Mexico, New York, North Dakota, Ohio, Oklahoma, Oregon, Pennsylva-nia, Rhode Island, Vermont, Washington, Washington D.C., and West Virginia.

Nine states plus the District of Columbia have legal recreational cannabis programs: Alaska, California, Colorado, Maine, Massachusetts, Nevada, Oregon, Vermont, Washington, and Washington D.C.

But it isn't just the medical benefits that are changing attitudes. There are serious social justice and financial issues that are forcing another look at our policies. One factor that should definitely not be overlooked when viewing our sorry history with cannabis is the human toll it has taken by imprisoning thousands of non-violent

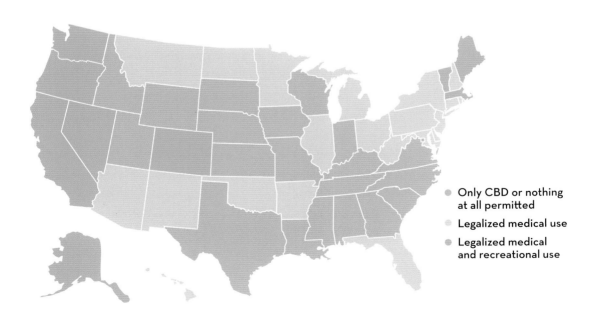

● Only CBD or nothing at all permitted

● Legalized medical use

● Legalized medical and recreational use

drug offenders, feeding the ever-hungry private prison system. Another shameful note is that people of color have been arrested, charged, and imprisoned at a rate of well over three times that of white Americans. Yet, usage rates between races is comparable. Furthermore, the amount of money devoted to drug enforcement is mind-boggling. In a June 2014 ACLU report, it was estimated that law enforcement spends over 3.6 billion dollars per year for marijuana possession alone! The report went on to say that someone is arrested for possession in the U.S. every 51 seconds (Wing 2016).

The lucrative private prison system is also to blame for mass imprisonment of cannabis users. Did you know that although the U.S. has about 5% of the world's population, that we house about 25% of the prison population (Gorman 2014)? Compared with other developed nations, such as the UK and Spain, we incarcerate more than seven times as many prisoners. Even compared with Russia, the U.S. incarcerates 75% more inmates. Clearly, our prison system churns out income and marijuana users are simple targets to fill beds and coffers. In 2015, according to an organization called Human Rights Watch, law enforcement made more than 500,000 arrests for simple cannabis possession for

personal use. The number of arrests for cannabis is nearly 15% higher than all arrests for violent crimes, including murder, rape, and serious assaults. Because the private prison system needs inmates to be profitable, as cannabis is legalized or decriminalized, the private prison system faces serious losses.

Legislation Worldwide

Of course, the U.S. is not the only nation figuring out how cannabis fits into the national landscape. A number of countries have already been experimenting with new legislation and innovative ideas. Let's look at a few of them.

Uruguay

Uruguay became the first nation to legalize cannabis in 2014. Popular leader Pepe Mujica spearheaded the efforts to legalize cannabis because Mujica wanted to stop the black market and because he believed in cannabis for health issues. The plan was to have adult citizens over the age of 18 register with a national registry. Once they registered, they could visit participating pharmacies and could purchase up to 40 grams of cannabis per month. 40 grams is roughly 1 ½ ounces, which is a lot of cannabis for most users to consume in a month. And this amount of cannabis was being sold at the bargain price of $1.30 per gram! For comparison's sake, if you were to walk into a Colorado dispensary, comparable product would cost six times as much (on sale). This bargain price was intentional, as it was thought this would cut out the black market.

After Mujica left office, it was left to Tabare Vasquez—an oncologist by trade—to institute the program. While there was widespread support among the population to put the program in place as soon as possible, Vasquez was dragging his feet because the idea of smoking cannabis challenged his training as an oncologist. But in the end, he relented, and a few pharmacies joined the program to popular delight.

In addition to being able to purchase cheap cannabis at pharmacies, Uruguayan citizens are also allowed to join cannabis-growing clubs that can grow up to 99 plants per year. Cannabis clubs are private "citizen only" entities that one pays an admission charge to join. The clubs grow cannabis together, split their harvest amongst members (and reportedly have great dinner parties). Although it looks like the overall program is rolling out smoothly—albeit slowly—a recent challenge is banking, which has caused pharmacies to slow enrollment in the program. We'll see how it all evolves,

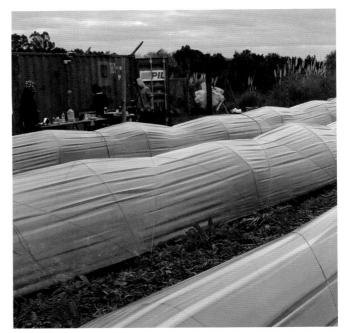

Join the club. In Uruguay, grow-club members grow up to 99 plants per year in greenhouse-like micro-tunnels.

but it appears that Uruguay will continue to be a cannabis trailblazer.

Other Countries of Latin America

Several Latin American countries, including Mexico, Brazil, Argentina, Chile, Colombia, and, most recently, Peru (CBD only) have legalized the use of medical cannabis; other countries in this region may follow suit soon. Mexico has also floated the idea of legalizing cannabis at resorts to induce tourism and to cut down on the illegal cannabis trade.

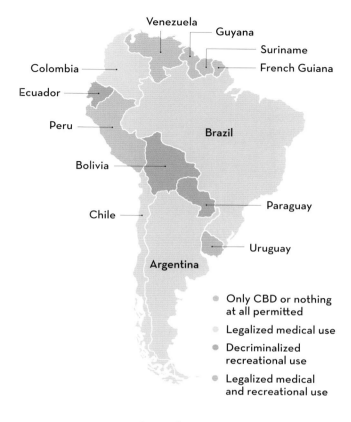

Venezuela
Guyana
Suriname
French Guiana
Colombia
Ecuador
Peru
Brazil
Bolivia
Chile
Paraguay
Argentina
Uruguay

- Only CBD or nothing at all permitted
- Legalized medical use
- Decriminalized recreational use
- Legalized medical and recreational use

Canada

As expected, Canada legalized recreational and medical cannabis for adult citizens (age 18 or 19 depending on the province) in summer 2018. The official date for the rollout of legal cannabis is October 17, 2018 and the world watches with great interest. This is a cannabis game changer, as Canada becomes the second country in the world (Uruguay was first) and the first member of the G-7 to legalize cannabis. Along with Australia, Canada has one of the highest cannabis

consumption rates in the world. When Justin Trudeau became Prime Minister, one of his announcements was that Canada planned to legalize both recreational and medical marijuana across all provinces. Initially, it was suggested that implementation could take place in summer 2018, but several law enforcement groups have asked to delay the program so they can better train their officers to handle issues such as citizens driving under the influence of cannabis. These voices were considered, but the momentum for legalization was too great to tolerate any major delays. As they roll out legalization, they realize that this means big business and a unique opportunity to carve out business opportunities for small, specialized producers and services. Through an innovative system of "micro-licensing," the following businesses will be given an opportunity to flourish:

- Small-scale growers
- Growers of starter materials, such as nurseries, that offer seeds, clones, and seedlings (starter plants)
- Industrial hemp growers
- Small scale micro-processors

Several of their larger cannabis companies are making deals to cross borders and are positioning their growers to export large quantities of

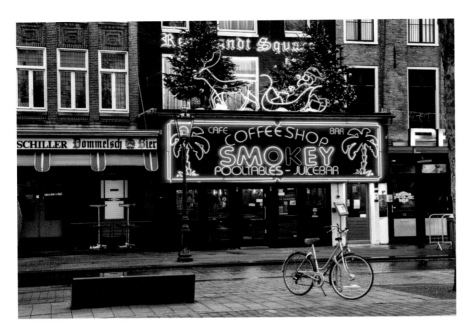

The streets of Amsterdam. Holland long ago decriminalized the consumption of cannabis, which has become an accepted part of the culture.

product. If they continue at this pace, Canada is likely to become a market leader in the cannabis world.

Europe

Germany already allows for medical cannabis and it is likely they will legalize cannabis soon. It is also notable that it looks like Germany will require insurance companies to pay for the medicine. Also, for users who do not have a medical prescription for medical cannabis, it is considered "self-harm" to use cannabis recreationally rather than a crime.

Switzerland has taken a purely economic approach; they are legalizing and taxing all THC products, regardless of potency. It is said that Austria may be inspired by this approach as well.

Spain has decriminalized the possession and use of marijuana, but it cannot be consumed in public. Because of a legal loophole, hundreds of private cannabis clubs have sprung up; these clubs must be non-profit and only serve adults. In part, because of their cannabis clubs, Spain is becoming a popular cannabis tourist destination.

Italy was slow to engage in the conversation about cannabis, but in an interesting twist, they have involved their military in the growth of medical cannabis. They want to stop the flow of cannabis from other nations and focus on growing high-CBD plants versus plants high in THC.

Holland allows for consumption of cannabis and hash (which is concentrated, pasty, high-THC cannabis) in "coffee shops" and currently possession of 5 grams or under has been decriminalized. This system has been in place since the '70s, but recently there has been a crackdown on public consumption (especially involving tourists) in border cities, such as Hague. Offenders are subject to a fine. It will also come as no surprise that some of the most knowledgeable underground growers have set up shop in Holland and some of the best seeds and cuttings are available here. This has happened because, strangely, although consumption is acknowledged and tolerated, it is technically illegal to grow cannabis in Holland. This is called their "backdoor problem"; some local mayors have allowed and encouraged small grow operations to supply product to "coffee shops." On a national level, there is pending legislation to allow for growers, but it is likely to take years before it passes.

Portugal has taken the novel approach of decriminalizing all drugs and they treat drug use as a medical/health issue and not a crime.

If anyone is caught with a 10-day supply of any drug (or less), they are referred to a treatment team who determines whether the user should go to treatment. The treatment team is composed of three people, namely a social worker, a psychiatrist, and an attorney. This small group, in consultation with the user, decides on small fines or free treatment options. Many users are simply fined and sent on their way.

The UK currently prohibits the use, growing, sale, or possession of cannabis. Law enforcement has leeway to issue a warning—generally if the user has 1 ounce or less—but if larger amounts are involved, fines and prison sentences are common. On the medical front, the UK is receiving pressure from patients, such as those afflicted with epilepsy, to be allowed to use cannabis. These grassroot pleas are being taken seriously, so we'll see if the UK changes policies regarding medical cannabis.

Eastern Bloc

Most countries in the Eastern Bloc have been slow to allow medical or recreational cannabis, though citizen's groups in favor of allowing medical marijuana are gaining traction. However, the Czech Republic and Poland now allow for the use of medical cannabis (but in the Czech Republic, cannabis is expensive and often has to be imported). On a more progressive note, Croatia and Macedonia have recently allowed cannabis for therapeutic uses and product is available in pharmacies. Serbia and Slovenia have recently legalized select cannabis products as well.

The Caribbean

The use and possession of cannabis in Puerto Rico and the U.S. Virgin Islands remains illegal (although in the Virgin Islands, possession of up to 1 ounce is decriminalized). In Jamaica, many visitors are surprised to learn that cannabis—though a major part of Jamaican culture and the Rastafarian religion—is technically illegal (but in practical terms, possession of small amounts is overlooked or taken care of with an official or "unofficial" fine). It is also likely that Jamaica and surrounding nations with strong tourist economies will legalize cannabis soon, as they are eyeing cannabis tourism to kick-start their economy. Other more conservative Caribbean nations, including Cuba, Barbados, and Dominica, simply consider cannabis to be illegal.

Australia/New Zealand

Australia has one of the highest rates of cannabis use in the world. It is estimated that over a third of adults 21 and older have used cannabis; Australia's native population has even higher use rates. In 2016, medical cannabis was legalized, and there is great momentum to legalize and regulate recreational cannabis as well; this movement is spearheaded by a large number of Australian cannabist activist groups. Individual states and territories enact and enforce their own unique regulations, which are largely focused on rendering small fines and recommending treatment options or simply taking a "live and let live" approach.

In New Zealand only synthetic cannabis formulated with THC and CBD by an approved pharmaceutical company is allowed for medical patients. But New Zealanders overwhelmingly support legalizing cannabis for adults and major change is expected in the short term.

Asia

Asia continues to have strict, even draconian, laws regarding cannabis. Except for Cambodia (where cannabis is becoming more and more popular with their youth to the point where it is consumed publicly) and India (where deep cultural traditions of various methods of consumption, such as the revered drink byang), enforcement of existing laws has become nearly impossible and certainly impractical.

Africa

South Africa is one of the largest cannabis growers in the world because the climate is well-suited to the plant. Only recently have South African government studies been commissioned to determine if cannabis should be partially legalized for medical issues. An important personal possession case in the courts was filed in March 2017, which could pave the way for private, personal use. The case was upheld, but still needs confirmed by the Constitutional Court and then an additional 24 months must pass in order for Parliament to enact legislation; but it looks like change is imminent.

Other African nations have declared cannabis illegal, but some don't truly pursue enforcement. However, a few interesting developments include:

- Lesotho, which borders South Africa, has long been a major grower and clandestine exporter to South Africa, but the government is looking to legitimize and regulate growers.
- In Morocco, cannabis remains illegal, but because such a large amount of hash is produced there, the government is exploring le-

galization and turns a blind eye to growing and modest consumption.

- Malawi's three main exports are fish, tea, and cannabis (also known as chamba) and the government takes a largely hands-off approach. A world-renowned high-sativa strain called Malawi Gold originates here and has become so popular that underground cannabis tourism is growing. In addition, Malawi is embarking on a pilot hemp-growing program.
- Ghana boasts a large number of users and public support for legalization, but governmental and religious agencies are offering stiff opposition.
- Swaziland has commissioned a government agency to study legalization. This has happened several times before, so it is uncertain if any changes will occur.

Antarctica

Antarctica technically has no governing body, but visitors and researchers must abide by the laws of their native land. However, there is no enforcement of these rules and a friend of mine who spent months there said many of the visitors find ingenious ways to bring cannabis with them. He created some very powerful clear tincture and simply brought it with him in a water bottle. It lasted him for months!

Profile

FOSTERING EQUALITY AND OPPORTUNITY

EBELE IFEDIGBO, *Co-Founder / Co-Executive Director, The Hood Incubator*

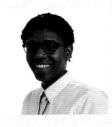

BY MARK COFFIN

Ebele Ifedigbo spearheads The Hood Incubator's business development and fundraising efforts. Ifedigbo is a Yale M.B.A. graduate committed to using business to foster innovation and racial equity in cannabis. Ifedigbo has served as an NAACP Economics Fellow, working to develop federal and state policies and programs aimed at closing the national Racial Wealth Divide. Ifedigbo's other professional experiences include working as a finance analyst at Ameriprise Financial, a legal and compliance summer analyst at Goldman Sachs, and an M.B.A. summer intern for worker cooperative development organization Project Equity. Ifedigbo received a joint B.A. in Economics and Philosophy with a minor in African Studies from Columbia University in New York City, and in June 2017 was awarded the highly competitive Echoing Green global social entrepreneurship fellowship on behalf of The Hood Incubator. In October 2017, Entrepreneur Magazine honored Ifedigbo as one of 2017's Most Daring Entrepreneurs, along with Jeff Bezos, Issa Rae, Elon Musk, and other global innovators. In November 2017, Ifedigbo was named to the 2017 Full Color 50 List and the 2018 Forbes 30 Under 30 List.

When I spoke with Ifedigbo, I asked what the drive was to become a part of the cannabis community.

At my core, I'm committed to Black people's economic freedom. From a young age, my dad would drive me around our low income Black neighborhood on the east side of Buffalo and passionately point out that the most prevalent businesses in the community—payday lenders, rent-to-own shops, check cash stores, and corner stores—often served to siphon much-needed economic resources out of the community rather than help it thrive. Seeing that dynamic first-hand, and later learning about the systemic realities of the racial wealth divide and how the drug war has contributed to fundamental economic disparities, catalyzed my passion for racial and economic justice.

In my career and academic endeavors, my guiding question has been, "Can business actually serve the ends of racial justice—if so, how?" While studying this question in business school, I had my ah-ha moment of realizing that the legalizing marijuana industry is the perfect opportunity to building economic and political power for Black communities and to repair the harms of the drug war. From then on, I hustled to figure out the best model for increasing Black participation in the industry, and that led to the creation of The Hood Incubator.

A final interesting note is that some nations export medical cannabis. They include Canada, Uruguay, the UK, and the Netherlands. Three additional nations that are likely to start exporting medical cannabis are Australia, Israel, and Colombia. Because it is such a lucrative crop, nations who import medical cannabis are likely to consider internal production soon.

The complicated history of this simple plant is certainly not over. The next decade will be a busy one for cannabis legislation, production, and products. Oh, and knowledge. We are going to learn a lot about this plant in the months and years to come.

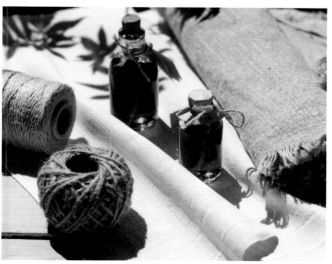

Hemp is amazingly versatile. While the consumption of parts of the marijuana plant has medical and recreational uses, other parts of the plant—usually referred to as hemp—can be used to create a wide variety of useful products.

Hemp

Technically, hemp, cannabis, and marijuana (oh my!) are not different. That is, hemp is cannabis and marijuana . . . and marijuana is cannabis and hemp. But hemp is only one type of cannabis and contains minor or trace amounts of THC. And marijuana is simply another word for cannabis, though most people have an image of an illicit drug with psychoactive properties when they hear the word marijuana.

Hemp is non-psychoactive and is an amazingly adaptable, valuable crop that was caught up in the prohibition of marijuana. We discussed the history of hemp and its place in American history, but here we will go into a bit more depth. Hemp is a plant, but it is also food and the basis for tens of thousands of products. It is one of the oldest crops that humans have cultivated, and you may recall that some reports have dated it back to 5000 B.C. in China. Around 500 B.C., the Greeks reported on the many uses of hemp—even touting its medicinal benefits. In medieval Europe, citizens cooked with hemp, using it in soup or as a filling for pies.

As the New World was being discovered, hemp was widely and regularly used on ships. In fact, the ropes on Columbus's ships were made of hemp. And artists such as Van

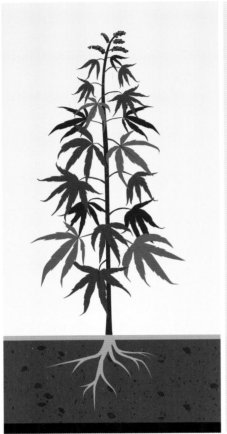

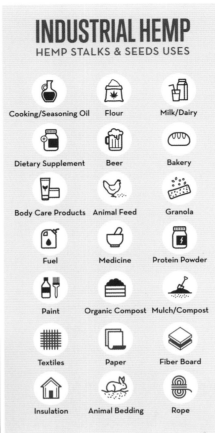

INDUSTRIAL HEMP
HEMP STALKS & SEEDS USES

Cooking/Seasoning Oil   Flour   Milk/Dairy

Dietary Supplement   Beer   Bakery

Body Care Products   Animal Feed   Granola

Fuel   Medicine   Protein Powder

Paint   Organic Compost   Mulch/Compost

Textiles   Paper   Fiber Board

Insulation   Animal Bedding   Rope

Building materials and beyond. Hemp can be used in a variety of manufacturing products, including building materials, the door panels of cars, poster board and many paper-type products, plastics, apparel, ethanol, carpeting, and a variety of health and beauty aids.

Gogh would paint on canvases that were blended from hemp and linen (Carbonnel 1980; "Painting Surfaces"). Also, as mentioned earlier, the Spanish brought hemp to the Americas in about 1545, and American colonists were required to plant hemp for England—they could even pay their taxes in hemp.

Like me, you are probably thinking, "With a history of so many beneficial uses and such wide acceptance, why is hemp use and growth even controversial in the U.S. today?" The answer is that many parts of the hemp plant were not distinguished from psychotropic cannabis, and under the Marihuana Act of 1937, it was made ridiculously expensive via an excessive tax. All of this means that hemp simply became too expensive to farm.

Hemp had a short-lived revival from 1942 to 1957, when the U.S. government encouraged farmers to grow

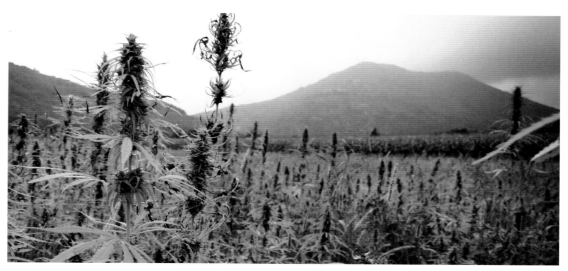

A viable crop for farmers. Hemp is a hearty crop that can be grown in a variety of soils and climates in almost all of the world.

hemp because of World War II. Since many resources were scarce, farmers were being asked to grow hemp for rope, canvas, and uniforms. There was even a campy movie that the government produced called *Hemp for Victory*. But once the war was over and the need for hemp had decreased, propaganda that tied hemp to its close cousin marijuana, began in earnest. Evocative journalism, combined with movies such as *Reefer Madness* and *Marijuana: The Devil's Weed* depicted marijuana as being responsible for wildly irrational behavior, accidents, and sexual promiscuity. Affected by damaging publicity and a decreasing market, by the late 1950s most hemp processors went out of business.

Even today, the hemp lobby is still trying to differentiate itself from other forms of cannabis. The U.S. attitude toward hemp is an anomaly: We are the only industrialized nation that prohibits the production of hemp (in nearly ⅓ of the country). But we can—and do—import hemp products and raw materials from many other countries, including China, the largest exporter of hemp and related products in the world.

Hemp can be used for everything from the door panels of cars to health and beauty aids, as well as one of the most popular products on the market today: hemp/CBD oil. Hemp is often confused with marijuana because they both come from cannabis plants, but hemp has no, or only trace amounts, of

Profile

CHAMPIONING FREEDOM FOR FARMERS

COURTNEY MORAN, *Hemp Attorney*

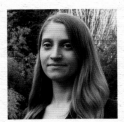

Courtney N. Moran, LL.M., founding principal of EARTH Law, LLC, found her passion for cannabis law reform after reading *The Emperor Wears No Clothes* by Jack Herer and Chris Conrad. While attending a plant biology class at Marquette University, her class assignment was to write a paper about a plant—Courtney chose cannabis and wrote about the environmental benefits it provides, verifying everything she learned from Jack's and Chris's book in scientific literature. Her advocacy never stopped. During law school at St. Thomas University, Courtney interned for Keith Stroup at NORML, and she now serves on the Board of Directors. Courtney continued to focus her education on industrial hemp, completing the world's first industrial hemp university course at Oregon State University, and focusing her Master of Laws in Environmental and Natural Resources Law program at Lewis and Clark Law School on Industrial Hemp Law, graduating magna cum laude. Since Courtney began her career, her firm, EARTH Law, LLC, remains dedicated to championing legal policy for a sustainable cannabis hemp industry.

Courtney has shared her passion through producing educational conferences during Hemp History Week, and founding the non-profits Oregon Hemp Industries Association and the Oregon Industrial Hemp Farmers Association. Courtney also had her law review article, "Industrial Hemp: Canada Exports, United States Imports" published in the *Fordham Environmental Law Review.*

Courtney has achieved momentous legislative strides in several states that passed legislation establishing industrial hemp as an agricultural commodity and providing for the foundation of industrial hemp programs. She continues to work to bring hemp legalization to states throughout the U.S., not only through strategic lobbying efforts but also as co-petitioner of the Relegalizing Industrial Hemp Project, a formal administrative rulemaking petition to the U.S. Drug Enforcement Agency that will remove industrial hemp from the Controlled Substances Act.

THC; most states mandate that hemp must contain less than 0.3% THC. It bears repeating: You cannot get high from hemp. But it does contain CBD, which has health benefits for many.

Hemp is also a viable, profitable crop for farmers because it is naturally pest resistant. It grows quickly, so it makes a great crop when rotating the fields, and some farmers have found it to be a

Do You Know Your Kush from Your Diesel?

Perhaps it is the spark of creativity that some of us feel when we partake but there is no denying that slang cannabis terms are a lot of fun to create and use. Which do you want to try?

Weed	Hash	Illy	M.J.	Garlic	Blaze
Tree	Crippy	Nugs	Fire	Spliff	Dime
Pot	Herb	Indo	Mook	Roach	Broccoli
Christmas	That Good-	Blunt	Mota	Hashish	Asparagus
Tree	Good	Mary Jane	Muggle	Shake	Bush
Grass	Chronic	Joint	Skunk	Hash	Zig-Zag
Shatter	Doobie	Ju-Ju	Purp Skurp	Yerba	Catnip
Dope	Dank	Fatty	Spliff	Dabs	Binger
Cocoa Puffs	Endo	Kaya	OG	Cabbage	Kief
Reefer	Bud	Loud	Trim	Green	Cheese
Scooby	Griefo	Kush	Parsley	Devil's Let-	Dutchie
Snacks	Flower	Indica	Vape	tuce	Cheddar
Ganja	Hydro	Leaf	Salad	Purple	
Scoobs	Nuggets	Sativa	Sticky Icky	Diesel	

good replacement for crops in decline, such as tobacco. To date, 33 states and Puerto Rico have introduced pro-hemp legislation, and 24 states have defined industrial hemp as distinct from other strains of cannabis. In addition, some states are allowing universities to team up with hemp farmers to produce hemp for research. Over the next few years, many of us feel that hemp will go back to its roots and once again become an accepted, appreciated crop across the nation.

DID YOU KNOW?

"Got to Get You into My Life" by the Beatles is about marijuana? In discussing his 1997 book, *Paul McCartney: Many Years to Come*, McCartney revealed that he wrote the song after being introduced to marijuana—and its many benefits—for the first time.

Chapter 2
THE SCIENCE OF CANNABIS

Let's spend a bit of time understanding what is in cannabis and understanding its active compounds. Cannabis is a group of plants that, as one of its nicknames suggests, grow like weeds. There are three main types of cannabis plants—*cannabis sativa* (suh-tee-vuh), *cannabis indica* (in-dik-uh) and *cannabis ruderalis* (roo-der-al-is). In addition, there are hundreds of hybrid cannabis plants that are blends of sativa, indica, and/or ruderalis plants. Today, the majority of cannabis plants by far are hybrids, but sativas and indicas are still very easy to find, with ruderalis being less common. There are hundreds of chemical compounds in cannabis, but we are going to focus on THC (tetrahydrocannabinol, pronounced tet-rah-hi-dro-kah-nab-i-nol) and CBD (cannabidiol, pronounced can-na-bid-e-all), the two compounds that are associated, respectively, with

being high and pain relief. It's worth exploring each of these plants and the compounds they contain so that you can understand the traits associated with each plant. There are hundreds of chemical compounds in cannabis; these are known as cannabinoids. Cannabinoids are simply the organic compounds that occur in the cannabis plant, such as THC, CBD, hemp oil, terpenes, and flavonoids (Watts 2006).

THC

THC is the chemical compound in cannabis that will give you a euphoric high. THC attaches to an element in your brain and surrounding tissues that impacts your perceptions. Some would say it alters your reality (usually for around 1 to 3 hours if smoked or vaped). An example of these exaggerated effects from pop culture would be the way the character Spicoli acts

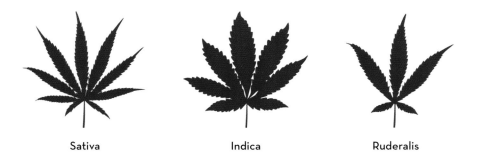

Sativa   Indica   Ruderalis

The basic plants. The three main types of cannabis plants are sativa, indica, and ruderalis. Hybrid varieties are often combinations of two or even all three types.

THC and CBD. The differing chemical makeup of THC and CBD make them appropriate for different uses. Though there are other cannabinoids present in cannabis, this book will only discuss THC and CBD.

NATURAL CANNABINOIDS

in *Fast Times at Ridgemont High* or any character in a Cheech and Chong movie. Of course, in the real world, THC can be helpful for pain management, sleeplessness, appetite stimulation, and relaxation.

CBD

CBD, on the other hand, is an active chemical compound found in the stalks, flowers, stems, resin, and seeds of cannabis plants that has analgesic, anti-inflammatory, and anti-anxiety properties that occur without making the user high. For many of us with

aches and pains, CBD attacks the inflammation in our bodies, allowing us to relax and sleep, thereby letting the body heal itself. Like ibuprofen, Tylenol, and Motrin, CBD reduces inflammation, but it does so naturally and apparently with no long-term consequences, while commercial analgesics are said to be taxing on the stomach, kidney, and liver over the long term.

Hemp oil, which is also known as CBD oil, is obtained by pressing hemp stalks, stems, flower, seeds, and resin and gathering the oil. It will not get you high and should not be confused with hash oil, which does contain THC and will give you the typical psychoactive effects. Some CBD products only contain oil from the seeds, which is not considered as effective as oil derived from the whole plant (called full spectrum or whole plant oil). Simply put, check the label to make sure you are getting more than hemp seed oil—which is not bad for you, but more like a good olive oil and much less like medicine. And the reason that you, as a consumer, can order CBD and hemp oil products and have them shipped to your home in any one of the 50 U.S. states is that the Farm Bill of 2014 defined hemp that contains less than 0.3% THC to be "industrial hemp"; that is what the various hemp and CBD oil products are made of ("2014 Farm Bill" 2014).

Before you run to order CBD products, let's take a minute to explain how CBD works in the body: welcome to the endocannabinoid system. This system was discovered by Israeli doctor and scientific researcher Raphael Mechoulam in the early '90s. Mechoulam is affectionately known as the Grandfather of Cannabis and he and his team are still hard at work today. Unlike the U.S., the Israeli government supports some cannabis research, so Mechoulam and his team have been

diligently working for over a quarter of a century (Mechoulam).

In 1992, Dr. Mechoulam and two researchers, Dr. William Devane and Dr. Lumir Hanus, discovered anandamide, a naturally occurring endogenous cannabinoid that most people know as the "runner's high" chemical. It is called anandamide after the Sanskrit word for "bliss." Further discoveries revealed the human body has a network of receptors in the brain and the body—now known as the endocannabinoid system. This system helps keep the body in balance by regulating many of the body's functions—such as blood sugar, hormones, immune functions, digestion, and regular heartbeat. Furthermore, it seems the endocannabinoid system communicates in two directions. Directions flow from the brain to the cells, and when cells are in distress, they send messages back to the brain. The system helps the body repair itself by reducing inflammation and protecting and repairing brain cells. In simplest terms, Mechoulam's work found that CBD and THC mirror the effects of anandamide.

There are two types of receptors: CBD1 are in the brain, organs, spinal cord, and surrounding tissue areas; CBD2 are in the immune systems. THC attaches to the CBD1 receptor, which is thought to be involved with

Profile

THE MIRACLE OF HOPE

TERRI LEEK and **JULIET FILLWEBER**, *Pure Hemp Collective*

Terri Leek and Juliet Fillweber are co-owners of the Pure Hemp Collective in Conifer, Colorado, which creates and sells a variety of cannabis products designed to relieve pain and treat a variety of medical conditions.

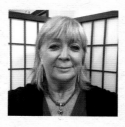

Terri Leek

My journey with cannabis remedies began when I was a child and my grandmother, Vina Bell, would make natural homemade plant products for the health of her family. I never thought that much of it as it was part of my everyday life. She grew a single hemp plant behind the garage by the rabbit hutches, where she used their droppings as fertilizer. Fast forward 40 to 50 years and I had moved to Colorado and was looking for relief for my own knee pain. I started making my own CBD salve and sharing it freely with friends and family. It became a phenomenon in our little town.

It was when I started sharing it that I began to see the miracle of that little molecule. Not only is it found in the cannabis/hemp plant, but in our bodies, as well as the bodies of all vertebrates. In fact, mother's milk is one of the richest sources of CBD. As a physiology teacher that says a lot to me. I have pictures of a client whose glial blastoma was so large that it covered one entire hemisphere of her brain. After using a bottle of 5,000mg tincture each month for three months, the tumor was reduced to the size of my thumb. MRIs don't lie. I am also happy to see the little things that it does, like reduce anxiety in children, pets, and adults. CBD is more than a passion for me: it is a mission.

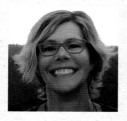

Juliet Fillweber

Hope is a funny thing, very elusive, hard to hang onto. In 2007, I lost all strength in my body, head to foot, tongue to toes. No explanation, just stillness; no movement, no energy. I was a young mom with passion and dreams, with success knocking on my door. I sat hopeless, unable to attain it.

After a diagnosis of a rare neuropathy, hope came in the form of CBD. Now I dream of sharing my education and life-changing CBD experiences. A plant given to the Earth to sustain us, to heal us, to bring hope. Now I spend my days formulating, blending, pouring, and selling CBD in every form—sharing with others the hope that all can change, that healing is here, real, and available to you.

Information is out there: keep reading; look for what you need; try new things. Be brave and step out to embrace what may be out of your comfort zone, and let those of us who have gone before you help pave the way.

pain, mood, emotions, coordination, appetite, and memories. This explains why THC affects the brain and the user feels high. CBD2, on the other hand, influences the immune system and affects inflammation and pain. CBD indirectly influences receptors around the body where the body is in distress. For example, if your knees are sore from playing tennis and you take CBD, the CBD will affect the receptors around the affected area and begin to battle inflammation. Apparently, the CBD receptors communicate in both directions, which means in our example that the affected knees "talk" to the brain and the brain responds to the knees. CBD also slows enzymes that break down our endocannabinoids, thereby increasing the body's natural levels of endocannabinoids. One of the primary benefits that inexperienced users of CBD often report is the additional benefit of better sleep. And as they are enjoying the sleep, CBD goes to work reducing inflammation and repairing the body.

Another intriguing study that Dr. Mechoulam conducted focused on concussions and the administration of CBD. Having noted CBD's neuro-protective capabilities regarding the brain, he hypothesized that concussion victims may benefit from an immediate large dose of CBD following injury. And given that Israel is a small country, Mechoulam was able to treat car crash victims within four hours of their accident; if concussion signs were visible, he administered CBD. As suspected, the CBD helped immensely and lessened or in some cases negated the effects of the concussion. Neighboring countries wanted to participate in the study as well. But when CBD was administered after 4 hours, the effect was minimal. These results suggest that time is of the essence when it comes to treating concussions. I can't help but think that sports leagues should take a close look at this study and explore the use of CBD for their athletes.

Mechoulam has also posited that there is an "Entourage Effect," which in simplest terms means that the whole cannabis plant works better as a unit for medicine than when segmented into parts. This means that he believes all parts of a cannabis strain should be used for medicine rather than just, say, the seeds, or breeding out CBD or THC. You may hear this called "full plant medicine." When ordering CBD or hemp oil products, I suggest looking for organic, whole plant or full-spectrum hemp; remember to note the potency (Brown 2011; Klein 2015).

COMMON TERPENES AND EFFECTS

Terpene Name	Aroma	Effects
Borneal	Spicy, menthol, camphor	Analgesic and anti-inflammatory
Carene	Sweet, cedar, pungent	Bone growth and calcium production
Caryophyllene	Spicy, warm, sweet, woody	Analgesic and anti-oxidant
Eucalyptol	Spicy, minty, camphor	Antibacterial and anti-inflammatory
Limonene	Sour, citrus	Anti-anxiety and anti-depressant
Pinene	Pine	Antibacterial and aids memory

Terpenes

Terpenes are the oils in cannabis that give it a distinct smell, such as mint, lemon, pine, or mushrooms. This is especially important in cooking, as some cannacooks and cannachefs like to pair particular cannabis strains with certain dishes. For example, if you cook with a strain with lemon profile, you may want to consider using it with fish or to brighten up a salad. But on the other hand, part of the expertise that cannacooks bring to the table is to mask or channel the pungent odor of cannabis so that a diner wouldn't even know cannabis was in a dish (but of course every responsible canna-cook tells their audience exactly what they are getting and what type of dose they are taking)! The chart above lists a few common terpenes, their distinct aroma, and effects.

Flavonoids

Flavonoids are the aromatic mole-cules that contribute to the overall taste of marijuana. That is, they con-tribute to the color, flavor, and smell of cannabis. Flavonoids are a huge family of compounds, and scientists have discovered more than 5,000 dif-ferent flavonoids. When the cannabis plant grows, flavonoids also help filter UV rays, repel pests, and inhibit the growth of fungus (Szalay 2015).

What is meant by a "strain?"

Now that we have a basic cannabis vocabulary—and tapping into our cursory knowledge of sativas, indicas, ruderalis, hybrids, and cannabis in general—we can turn our attention to the wonderful, ever-growing world of cannabis strains. Would you believe that there are easily over 500 differ-ent strains and new strains are being developed every day? The amount

Profile

DOPE INFORMATION FOR THE CANNABIS COMMUNITY

JAMES ZACHODNI, *Co-Founder and Chief Creative Officer of* DOPE *Magazine*

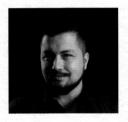

I published my first magazine in 2007. Hard to imagine then that starting a simple lifestyle and fashion magazine in Seattle would lead me to founding *DOPE Magazine* and seeing it grow to the heights it has reached thus far.

When my good friend (and current partner at *DOPE*) David Tran decided to invest into a small medical cannabis dispensary back in 2010, it quickly opened my eyes to a whole new industry that was being formed right before me. The only issue I saw was the lack of information out there for people to learn about cannabis, or where to advertise their fledgling cannabis businesses. Since David knew that my partner and I were magazine publishers, he approached us to put together a magazine about the medical cannabis industry. We agreed.

We quickly put our heads down and came up with the name DOPE and subsequently the acronym for it: Defending Our Patients Everywhere. It had a nice ring. We then needed a national platform to launch our magazine and saw that Hempfest, the world's largest cannabis festival, was a short 60 days away

and right in our backyard. We had to make the deadline to launch at Hempfest.

The feat was not impossible since we had years of experience publishing magazines, but one thing we didn't have was someone for the cover who would be impactful enough to have on our inaugural issue. We dug deep into our contact list and found out we had a contact to the Mayor of Seattle at the time, Mike McGinn, who was a big medical cannabis proponent. He agreed to be on our cover.

The rest, I guess you can say, is history. We battled the August sun to personally hand out 10,000 magazines at Hempfest that year and the press we received from having the Mayor on our cover was far-reaching. Within months after launching, *DOPE* became a household name with Washington cannabis enthusiasts and we began telling all the important stories that were forming daily, from social justice issues to the impending legalization of Washington and Colorado. *DOPE* is now the largest free cannabis publication (currently in 27+ states and Canada) and prints 150,000 copies monthly.

I will never forget how symbiotically my experience in magazine publishing and the stories of the emerging cannabis industry came together to form something that truly is DOPE.

of THC and CBD, the flavor, and the potency changes from one strain to the next, so knowing the benefits of each will help you manage your expectations and medical or recreational needs.

Let's talk more about sativa, indica, and hybrid cannabis strains. Sativa plants are tall and skinny with thinner, longer leaves. Sativa is known for energy, creativity, and focus. Indica plants are short and fat, with broader leaves. Indica is often used for relaxation and sleep. Ruderalis originated in Eastern Europe and Russia. It is much smaller than the other plants, but can contain high amounts of CBD, which makes it an inviting source of hemp oil. Ruderalis also "auto-flowers," meaning it blooms predictably, with age rather than because of light cycles.

The story of how cannabis was originally classified goes back to scientist Carl Linnaeus, who you may remember from your high school biology class as the Father of Taxonomy. Over his lifetime, Linnaeus named more than 10,000 lifeforms, including *Cannabis sativa L* in 1753. The letter L stands for Linnaeus, since he was the first person to name it. And when he did name it, he thought it was a single species. But roughly thirty years later, another scientific luminary, Jean-Baptiste Lamarck, identified a second cannabis species: *Cannabis indica Lam* (for Lamarck). Then, in the twentieth century, a group of Russian scientists identified a third species: *Cannabis ruderalis*. These terms are the same naming conventions that we use today (Watts 2006).

Today, a large percentage of cannabis strains are hybrids. Hybrids are constantly being created as growers attempt to magnify the best effects of the many strains available. Hybrids are also produced via cuttings and grafting, which accelerates the grow process. According to some growers, nearly every cannabis plant exhibits some evidence that it is at least part hybrid—to the point that now a more useful designation between plants may be thin leaf versus broad leaf.

A handful of heirloom or landrace cannabis strains have also been found. These are the "original" strains, such as Afghani (an indica strain) and Durban Poison (a sativa strain), and they are often used to create hybrids. For example, the Afghani strain's profile appears in most hybrids that are indica dominant. As with plants like heirloom tomatoes, there are growers who are trying to preserve landrace plants and seeds.

Among some growers, there is an emphasis on creating the most powerful THC strains, because that is what

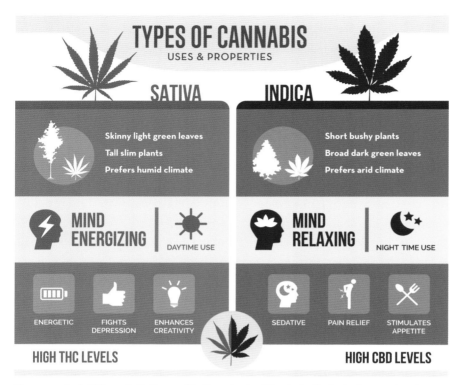

The same but different. Sativa and indica plants differ in both their chemical makeup and their appearance, but most of what is available commercially is a hybrid strain that has characteristics of each.

some users are after—and will pay a premium for this. On the other hand, as noted, there is also interest in preserving landrace strains or in creating high-CBD strains. And somewhere in the middle, there are master growers who are creating boutique strains that deliver specific benefits—such as helping the user sleep, stimulating appetite, or enabling more focus.

There could easily be a separate book written about cannabis strains, but it's not necessary for most users. A simple overview will turn up a list of popular strains that many dispensaries carry. If you want to do further research on your own, Leafly.com and cannabist.co are great sources to browse and learn about strains.

Sativa

Sativa dominant strains are often considered the more social variety of cannabis, and they play an integral role in an infused dinner party. Sativa is associated with energy, creativity, concentration, laughter, and heightened senses. If cannabis is consumed during the daytime, it is likely a sativa strain. Common examples of sativa strains are:

- Sour Diesel
- Blue Dream
- Super Silver Haze
- Jack Herer
- Super Lemon Haze
- Purple Haze
- OG Sour Diesel
- Durban Poison
- Maui Waui

Indica

Indica strains are associated with relaxation, sleep, and lessening of anxiety. Indica is often consumed after work or at bedtime. Humorously, when it is especially potent, it's sometimes referred to as "in-da-couch"; mostly, it often just helps people relax or relieves their pain. Common examples of indica strains are:

- Granddaddy Purple
- Northern Lights
- OG Kush
- Master Kush
- Afghani
- Purple Urkel
- G-13
- Hindu Kush
- Hashplant
- Chronic

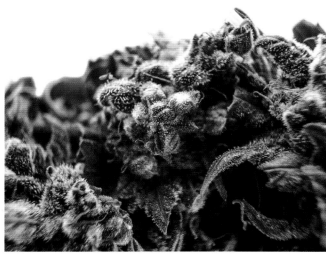

A high-THC bud. Buds of plants high in THC are resiny and sticky.

Sticky bud. Under a magnifying glass, you can see the trichomes, which look like pale white golf balls on tees.

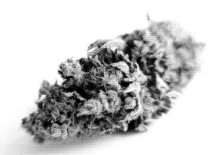

Hybrid

Hybrid strains, as you might expect, combine sativa, indica, ruderalis, or any or all of the above. The reason growers create hybrids is to capture the best elements of different strains. So, for example, they may be attempting to create a strain that makes the user feel full of energy or will help them sleep. Examples of popular hybrid strains include:

- White Widow
- AK-47
- Blueberry
- Purple Kush
- Pineapple Express
- Strawberry Cough
- NYC Diesel
- Bubble Gum
- Juicy Fruit
- Purple Skunk

CBD

CBD strains are especially beneficial for consumers who have medical issues but do not want to experience any high or heightened anxiety. Be aware that these strains do contain some THC, so we have listed the approximate ratio of CBD to THC for you as well (Seppa 2010, 16–20). If you are new to using cannabis, you may want to start with a very high CBD/low THC strain and then work your way towards a 1:1 ratio, which reportedly works well for many. And if you are too nervous to take this step, stick with CBD and hemp oil products.

Here then, are some popular CBD-dominant strains:

- Ringo's Gift 24:1
- ACDC 20:1
- Harle-Tsu 18:1
- Stephen Hawking Kush 5:1
- Cannatonic 3:1
- Harlequin 5:2
- Canna-Tsu 1:1
- Pennywise 1:1
- Sour Tsunami 1:1
- Sweet and Sour Widow 1:1

How Cannabis Is Grown

There are four ways cannabis is commercially grown. This will give you some insight in case you would like to grow your own cannabis, which some states allow.

Cannabis is primarily grown for commercial use in one of four ways:

- Indoors with artificial lights and with light given at calculated intervals;
- In a greenhouse with artificial lights and with lights on timers;
- In a greenhouse using the sun;
- Outdoors using natural sunlight.

Cannabis that is grown indoors is usually on the expensive side, but because it was grown in a controlled environment, it is often more potent, denser, and free of pests and pesticides. If cannabis is grown outdoors, it is cheaper to grow because it uses

Indoor growing. In less-ideal climates or for year-round growing under manageable conditions, greenhouses with timed lighting and watering systems can be highly efficient.

The old-fashioned way. Farming cannabis outdoors like traditional crops is common in areas where it is allowed by law.

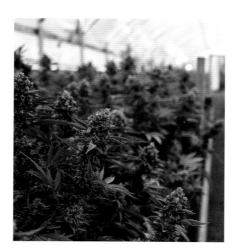

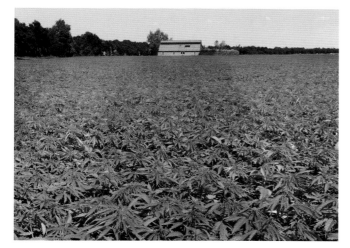

Homegrown

First, get to know your state regulations. You may only be allowed to grow a certain number of plants. Seedlings, immature plants, and mature plants may have individual limitations depending on the state. Keep in mind that you certainly won't be able to sell any cannabis you grow, and there may be further regulations such as keeping plants out of public sight. But interestingly, many states allow you to "gift" up to an ounce of your homegrown product—instead of "Puff, Puff, Pass," it's more like "Grow, Grow, Gift"!

You have several options if you'd like to home grow. You can plant your cannabis seed in the spring, and if all goes well, your harvest will come in in the fall. This assumes that you are growing outside and using natural sunlight. If you decide to grow indoors, you will need to invest in lights on a timer. The reason that lights are so important is that once your mature plant is exposed to 12 hours of light and 12 hours of dark, this will trigger the growth of buds.

This is assuming you are growing a (primarily) sativa or indica strain. Ruderalis seeds are much harder to find, and you would only grow those if you wanted a strain high in CBD. Plus, the yield of ruderalis is modest at best,

natural sunlight, and the buds are fluffier. Greenhouse cannabis is somewhere in the middle; this method uses natural sunlight and less water. You should also look for organically grown weed. It takes more attention and expertise, but you avoid chemicals and pesticides.

but it would be an educational experience to grow. You may recall that ruderalis flowers after a predictable amount of time has passed, rather than being forced to flower because of 12 hours of light and 12 hours of darkness.

Instead of growing cannabis from seed, a more popular and easier method is to purchase a small cannabis plant, called a seedling or sometimes a clone, at a dispensary. This will ensure that you have a healthy plant and a strain that you prefer. If you invest in a small plant, make sure to find out what kind of nutrients your plant may need over time—and when to give it the nutrients—how much light and darkness it will need, how long it will need to grow, and how to

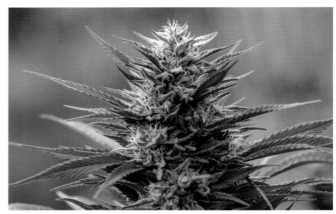

A different kind of cola. The single large bud on top of a marijuana plant is the most potent part of the plant, and it is referred to as a cola.

repel pests. Fortunately, there are many, many books, photos, and videos to help you. From the home growers I've spoken to, one of the keys seems to be to learn as you go. That is, a little bit of experience goes a long way and the only way to get that experience is to try to grow a plant.

Simple Instructions for a Single Homegrown Plant

To get you started, here is a little grow primer. We will not discuss subtleties like planting cuttings or trimming to increase the number of buds that flower. I think it is valuable to see how a cannabis plant normally grows; you will end up with a single large bud on top called a "cola." It's like a dense pine cone and it will be the most potent part of the plant. As you gain

DID YOU KNOW?

The Marijuana Policy Project's list of the *Top 50 Most Influential Americans to Use Marijuana* included Bill Gates, Presidents Barack Obama and George W. Bush, Michael Bloomberg, Richard Branson, Oprah Winfrey, Clarence Thomas, George Clooney, Tom Brokaw, Martha Stewart, LeBron James, Sanjay Gupta, Stephen Colbert, and other notables of the political, business, and art arenas?

experience, you will learn how to get additional plants from a single mother and how to maximize yield. But let's start with a simple method. Finally, here is a bit of trivia for you: it is only the female plants that produce bud. So, if you home grow, throw away your males and keep your females separate so they won't be pollinated, because that's the only way they'll produce bud. To identify male plants look for tiny balls (no kidding) where the leaves attach to the stem. Conversely, female plants will have wispy hairs where the leaves attach to the stem.

Now back to planting:

1. You need a breathable pot with good drainage.
2. Use organic soil with nutrients.
3. Allow the plant to mature for at least 4 to 6 weeks before triggering flowering.
4. To keep the plant from flowering during the growth period, keep it in direct sunlight/light for 18 to 20 hours a day.
5. Once mature, trigger flowering by changing the light schedule to 12 hours in direct light and 12 hours in absolute darkness.
6. For lighting, put the plant in sunlight or under a 250-watt bulb with an HID lamp from your local hardware store.
7. Water if the soil feels dry when you feel about an inch down, but it's better for the soil to be slightly dry then overly wet.
8. Cannabis plants seem to like only slightly moist soil, and temperatures in the mid 60s, 70s, and 80s.
9. You will want to harvest (or at least take your plant inside) when temperatures at night consistently dip down into the 40s; do not expose your plant to frost!
10. For more advice on home growing, visit cannabist.co, and good luck.

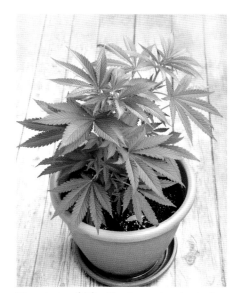

The circle of life. Plants can be started from seed indoors and transplanted, just like many other plants you find in the garden.

If you grow outdoors, here are a couple simple tips to keep pests away from your plants naturally. Consider planting basil, rosemary, marigolds, and clover next to your plants. The basil, rosemary, and marigolds will naturally repel pests, and clover is beneficial to the soil. You can also put ladybugs on your cannabis plant and the ladybugs will eat the pests, but you need to do this at the beginning of the grow season.

Harvesting

If you have successfully grown a cannabis plant, you will want to harvest it when it is at its most resiny. That is, if you use a magnifying glass, you will see a bunch of sticky, white, miniature balls that look like Christmas lights covering the bud and leaves. When your plant is on a 12 hours of light and 12 hours of dark cycle, monitor your plant daily; when it looks like most of the bud and surrounding leaves are covered in Christmas lights, you are ready to harvest. This is usually about 2 weeks after the 12 and 12 light pattern begins.

When you harvest, you can either cut the entire plant a couple of inches above its roots, or you can cut individual buds right next to the stalk. Leave a good amount of the stem or at least about an inch with individual buds to hang them upside down in a well-ventilated room for about a week

DID YOU KNOW?

The DEA's own Chief Administrative Judge ruled cannabis should be reclassified under Federal Law? In his 1988 remarks in The Matter of Marijuana Rescheduling, Judge Francis L. Young stated that "Marijuana, in its natural form, is one of the safest therapeutically active substances known to man. By any measure of rational analysis marijuana can be safely used within a supervised routine of medical care. It would be unreasonable, arbitrary and capricious for DEA to continue to stand between those sufferers and the benefits of this substance..."

to 10 days to give the plant time to dry a bit. A simple method is to hang a string across the room and then use a clothespin to hold the stem of the bud on the line.

Once the hanging buds or entire plant are partially dried (they should still feel spongy but don't touch them too much or you'll remove some of the resin/potency), you will be ready to trim the surrounding "sugar" leaves—the surrounding leaves gently touch the bud, and these leaves do have some potency, but not as much as the buds themselves. Place a piece of cardboard or poster board on a

Tending to the plants. These plants are drying and will be ready to be trimmed soon.

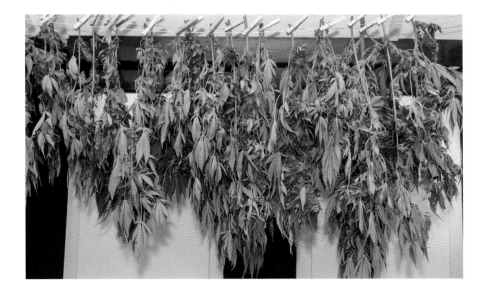

large, flat surface, hold an individual bud by the stem, and using small sharp scissors like nail scissors, trim the leaves closely, but do not cut/trim the bud. Place the trimmed bud in a sealed glass jar and store in a cool, dark place. Place the trimmings, or what is known as shake, in a glass jar as well. Trimmings work well for infused cannabis cooking, which we will get to on page 92. Repeat this process until all buds are trimmed and jarred.

Once all the buds and shake are in jars, a couple times a day open the jars (this is called "burping" because of the smell) and let air naturally circulate around the bud for 15 to 20 minutes. After a few days, or possibly a week depending on your climate and air circulation, your bud will be ready to smoke, make edibles with, and more. Congratulations; you've done it! You've grown your own!

A final word about growing your own cannabis plant is to mention that you should strongly consider getting your bud tested. Whether you are raising cannabis for medical purposes or for recreation, wouldn't you like to know what you are consuming? In some cases, your health may depend on it. There are labs in your state that will test your bud and can tell you how much CBD and/or THC it contains (potency), if there is any mold or pests present, and more. There are also some home testing kits available, but some of them are ridiculously difficult to use, so read product reviews and look for videos on how to use the kits.

Chapter 3

MEDICAL CANNABIS

I mentioned that one reason for renewed interest in cannabis is the potential medical benefits. With the opioid crisis hitting a fever pitch, people suffering from a number of chronic conditions, as well as temporary pain, are looking for natural alternatives. Cannabis is one of those alternatives and for some people, it is a literal life-saver.

Some of you may have heard of a very popular cannabis strain that is often made into tinctures or drops called Charlotte's Web. In fact, it may be one of the most publicized strains and products available; here is the story behind it. A little girl named Charlotte had epilepsy so severe that she was having seizures nearly every day. Her parents, at their wits' end, contacted the Stanley Brothers in Colorado, who had been developing some healthy hemp oil products. They set to work, and soon crossbred a strain high in CBD and low in THC now called Charlotte's Web that helped her condition immensely. Charlotte went from having a seizure a day to only having a couple seizures per year. So now we have a cannabis strain called Charlotte's Web that is widely used to create hemp oil to treat many conditions, including epileptic seizures.

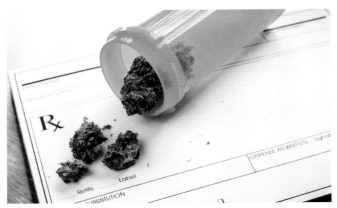

Medical uses abound. A variety of long- and short-term medical conditions can be treated successfully with medical marijuana.

It is stories like Charlotte's that have moved the medical cannabis conversation forward. Patients with painful conditions, such as multiple sclerosis, Lou Gehrig's disease, AIDS, PTSD, and more have demonstrated that cannabis can help their condition. State agencies are beginning to take notice and are slowly but surely embracing the use of medical cannabis.

What Conditions Are Covered by Medical Marijuana?

In the U.S., more and more states are legalizing medical cannabis, with roughly two-thirds of the states allowing for legal medical marijuana— something unthought-of not too long ago. Each state has their own list of qualifying medical conditions, but the most common conditions include:

- Epilepsy
- Multiple sclerosis (and other related muscle spasticity conditions)
- Cancer
- Chronic pain, including wasting syndrome
- Glaucoma
- HIV/AIDS
- Hepatitis C
- ALS, a.k.a. Lou Gehrig's disease
- Crohn's disease
- Post-traumatic stress disorder
- Conditions that are covered in a few states include Tourette's syndrome, severe arthritis and fibromyalgia, Alzheimer's, autism, ulcerative colitis, anxiety, and sleep apnea.

A resource that may be of use if you are researching cannabis as medicine is Michael Backes' book titled *Cannabis Pharmacy: The Practical Guide to Medical Marijuana*. What is truly impressive is his coverage of conditions. For each of the following health challenges, Backes offers a brief introduction, covers historical uses, discusses proper dosage, details methods of ingestion, suggests particular strains, and gives cautions and tips. If you have one of the following conditions or are researching for a loved one, this book would a good place to start:

- Alzheimer's disease
- Anxiety disorders
- Arthritis
- Asthma
- Attention deficit hyperactivity disorder (a.k.a. ADHD)
- Autism spectrum disorder
- Autoimmune disorders
- Cachexia (a.k.a. wasting disorder) and appetite disorders
- Cancer
- Chronic fatigue syndrome
- Diabetes
- Fibromyalgia
- Gastrointestinal disorders
- Gerontology (pain/arthritis, appetite issues, and sleeplessness)
- Glaucoma
- Hepatitis C
- HIV/AIDS
- Insomnia and sleep disorders
- Migraines and headaches
- Multiple sclerosis and movement disorders
- Nausea and vomiting
- Neuropathy
- Pain (this is the most popular condition for which cannabis is used)
- Parkinson's disease
- Post-traumatic stress disorder
- Schizophrenia
- Seizure disorders
- Skin conditions

A few other helpful topics covered after these conditions include "Cannabis and Adolescence," "Cannabis and Children," "Cannabis and Pregnancy," "Cannabis and Preventive Medicine," "Cannabis and Women's Health," and "Cannabis Dependency and Withdrawal." Overall, the information is interesting, clear, and provides good starting points for research and use.

What Is the Difference Between Medical and Recreational Cannabis?

Medical cannabis and recreational cannabis can be the same end product, but which part of the plant is used, how it is cultivated, how it is dosed, and how it is consumed is where the difference lies. Depending on the condition one is trying to

Profile

CHANGING LIVES

MITCH MEYERS, *Dispensary Owner, Cultivator, and Patient Advocate*

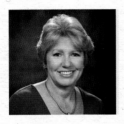

I spent 10 years honing my skills in marketing and brand development with Anheuser-Busch. I left for an entrepreneurial opportunity to start a marketing agency with a creative director. We built a wonderful agency and sold it, so I could retire young. I bought a second home in Colorado and befriended a woman who was a "caregiver" in the Colorado medical market. I saw her successfully treat cancer, Crohn's disease, epilepsy, and chronic pain. In many cases, she gave people their lives back. This was my "ah-ha" moment about cannabis. It is an amazing plant, put on this planet for a reason. Our government has systematically lied and misled us for political and financial reasons to keep it federally illegal. I began researching for hours and months on end and got even more indignant about the research that truly exists about its benefits (never mind that our government slyly patented cannabinoids in 1999 for medical purposes). Then, there is the social injustice....

I led a team in Illinois to get a dispensary license in 2014. I applied for and received a cultivation and dispensing license in Missouri in 2015. I hear families say every week, "You saved our son's/daughter's life." I didn't. The plant did. How can this simple solution not be available to everyone? It is un-American.

I am now operating in three more states with dogged determination to bring this to as many people as possible. So much for those retirement plans!

States that Recognize Other States' Cannabis Cards

These states are:
Arizona, Hawaii, Maine, Michigan, Nevada, New Hampshire, Rhode Island, and Pennsylvania.
In Pennsylvania, the only reciprocity applies to adults who have medical cannabis product for a minor. Also, most of the states will not allow you to purchase product at a medical dispensary, but you will not be penalized if you are carrying small amounts of cannabis. If you need your cannabis for a medical condition while traveling, the best advice is to visit a legal recreational cannabis state.

treat, different products, different THC and/or CBD potencies, different consumption methods, and particular doses are employed. Medical patients, in consultation with their physicians, often have to consider rate of absorption, how much medicine will be delivered to their body, and if they are limited to particular ingestion methods. For example, a patient may have trouble swallowing pills, so they may look to smoking, vaping, topicals, or suppositories. Each of these methods provides some benefits and challenges, but the good news is that more and more options are available and the creativity in this market shows no evidence of slowing.

In practical terms, medical patients may have access to products that are not available to recreational users and medical cannabis products are often less expensive than recreational products. An example of a different approach to medical versus recreational cannabis is that, until recently, medical patients in Oregon had access to one part of a dispensary and recreational users were led to another part of the dispensary. Recreational users could only look longingly at edibles and tinctures as their choices were limited to flower/bud. And in New York, medical patients could not buy flower at a dispensary because of a long-lasting no-smoking campaign. So be sure to check your state's requirements, spend time with a qualified doctor to acquire your medical cannabis card, and always carry your card with you for legal protection and possible product discounts. There are some states who offer reciprocity when it comes to medical cannabis, which means if you travel to another state, you may still be able to get your medicine.

On the recreation side, users often gravitate to smoking cannabis (with dozens and dozens of strain choices), vaping, or using edibles (infused cannabis treats). Edibles and infused beverages are increasing in popularity and feature inviting products like infused gummies, chocolates, ice cream, and fruity infused drinks. The portability, discreetness, and long-lasting effects all contribute to the popularity of edibles. In fact, I know many friends who fly after taking an edible and report that it made the trip faster and more pleasant.

What Is Synthetic Marijuana?

Not surprisingly, several pharmaceutical companies have developed and are developing synthetic versions of cannabis. The reason for this is simple. Doctors can prescribe these synthetic drugs and insurance companies will pay for them. Two of the most popular synthetics that you may have heard of are Marinol and Sativex. Marinol, which was introduced in 2004, is similar to cannabis that is high in THC. It is a gel capsule used for medical conditions like HIV/AIDS and cancer. Weirdly, it is listed as a Schedule III substance even though it is similar to cannabis and is legal in the U.S. Sativex, on the other hand, is a pepperminty spray that consists of a 1:1 CBD to THC formula and is taken orally. The most common condition for which Sativex is prescribed is MS and related muscle spas-

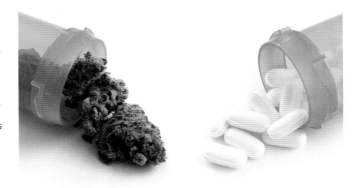

From the lab. Synthetic versions of marijuana are now available as an alternative to medical cannabis and in areas where medical cannabis is illegal.

ticity. But the maker of Sativex, GW Pharmaceuticals, are hoping that it will eventually be approved for diabetes, schizophrenia, epilepsy, and cancer as well. Unlike Marinol, Sativex is not yet legal in the U.S., though it is legal in 30 other countries.

What Is CBD?

If you have been reading the news, even as a casual observer, you have probably heard the abbreviation CBD and its potential as powerful, effective medicine. CBD (cannabidiol—pronounced canna-bid-e-all) is a major component in cannabis (along with THC—pronounced tetra-hydro-canna-bid-e-nall)—the difference is that CBD will not make the user feel high. That is, it is not psychoactive.

CBD is composed of the hemp plant's seeds, stalks, leaves, and stem, and by law must contain less than 0.3% THC (in most states). So, it is legal and available for purchase in all 50 states. One thing I learned very quickly is that you must learn how to read labels in this market. Common sense may tell you that one serving of an infused beverage should be 12 ounces as it is with beer, soft drinks, seltzer and the like. But check the label; it may be 2, 4, or even 6 servings. Also, the words "hemp" and "CBD" are used interchangeably.

Why Is CBD Legal?

In part, we have the Farm Bill of 2014 and great public interest in the health benefits of CBD to thank for CBD's (mostly) legal status and for the start of the revitalization of the industrial hemp industry. In general terms, the difference between hemp and psychoactive cannabis is the amount of THC resin that the plant produces (but note that there are high-resin cannabis plants that only contain a modest amount of THC but do contain impressive amounts of CBD). Some growers argue that industrial hemp is not the best source of CBD and that we should use high-resin/high-CBD oil from the whole cannabis plant, but for now it is one of the few options we

have. There is also strong belief that THC and CBD work best together but again, for now, only CBD is allowed in many states.

As with many aspects of cannabis, there are subtleties when you say something is legal, and the take on CBD is no different. While most would agree that the 2014 Farm Bill allows for the free sale of CBD and hemp oil across the nation, it is still considered a Schedule 1 drug, so some would deem it illegal. There is also the issue of crossing state lines. Take Colorado for example: It is legal to grow hemp in Colorado and, in fact, Colorado leads the nation in hemp production. Therefore, if you are a Colorado citizen, you can legally buy Colorado-grown CBD and hemp oil. But if you are in a neighboring state, you are not supposed to be able to buy Colorado CBD, because it would have to cross state lines—and cannabis is never supposed to cross state lines. To muddy the issue further, we have been importing hemp products from other nations for decades. If you order CBD online, you may receive product from China, Canada, and Latin America (and hemp seeds from France); this is perfectly legal. One bright spot is that there is legislation in the House of Representatives now that would legalize hemp nationwide.

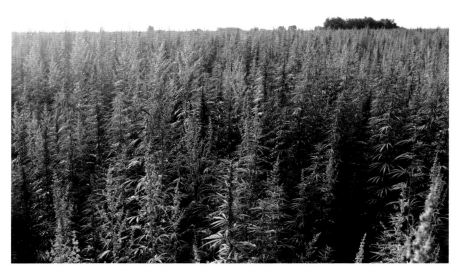

Whole plant products use just that. Different parts of the plant are used for different uses, but CBD products labeled "whole-plant" use all parts of the plant.

A strong advocate of the bill is Mitch McConnell, because his state of Kentucky would benefit greatly as hemp is a perfect replacement for the down-trending tobacco farms.

With CBD gaining a reputation as useful, natural medicine that treats inflammation, it should come as no surprise that the CBD oil or hemp oil have become very popular products. But like most products, caveat emptor (let the buyer beware)—make sure if you are purchasing CBD products that they are made from the entire hemp plant and not merely from hemp seeds. If you use hemp seed oil, you are getting cheaper oil with limited medical effects. That is, hemp seed oil is more like a good olive oil and that applies to raw hemp seeds

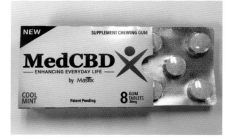

Check for dosage info. Packaging on CBD products, such as this gum, lists the potency (or milligrams per dose); for example, the CBD gum in the photo is 10 mg per piece.

as well—they are healthy, but they are not medicine. On the other hand, full-spectrum hemp oil, which uses all parts of the plant, can provide CBD and pain relief. Also, note that the term "CBD oil" is used interchangeably with "hemp oil." Once you determine that you are getting hemp oil and not merely hemp seed oil, be sure to pay attention to the potency of the product and follow your doctor's recommendations regarding dosing.

How Do I Find a Cannabis Doctor?

If you are interested in exploring the medical possibilities of cannabis, you'll want to start by researching the qualifying conditions of your state and talking with your doctor. Also, note that some states only allow CBD drops/tinctures to be used and do not allow the use of any THC (the part that gets you high) product. Of course, your doctor may not be sympathetic toward nor knowledgeable about cannabis. Don't let this thwart

Profile

SELF-ADVOCACY DURING HEALTH CHALLENGES

ANDREA DOW, *Self-Advocacy and Wellness: My CBD Journey*

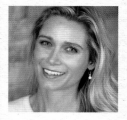

I am passionate about self-advocacy and personal empowerment in the face of health challenges. Being diagnosed with Hodgkin's lymphoma as a teenager and then thyroid cancer in my twenties, I am intimately familiar with the journey from fear and despair to recovery and vitality.

I was halfway through my 24 chemotherapy treatments for Hodgkin's when I was introduced to cannabis. The twelve treatments that I had already had were really taking a toll on my body, and I had 12 more to go. My body was withering away, my hair and appetite were completely gone, my bones ached, and I could no longer keep food down. My brother suggested that we consider cannabis. Legal or not, my parents did not flinch at the idea in hopes that it would provide some relief in a situation that left them paralyzed with helplessness.

Cannabis provided incredible relief to me during that time so many years ago. It relieved a lot of the pain and helped with nausea and appetite, which allowed me to regain strength and stamina. The imprint this experience had on me was life-changing. I experienced first-hand the relief cannabis can provide to people who are suffering.

Over time, I have become an advocate for my own healing. Extensive lifestyle changes through nutrition, movement, and meditation have helped significantly, and I continue to move toward a wellness perspective that relies on the healing properties of nature. As such, I have begun yet another phase by uncovering the healing effects of cannabidiol (CBD). Spending most of my time scouring articles and research studies, I am optimistic about the potential that CBD has in our wellness future. Months ago, I could not even pronounce cannabidiol. Now, I have made CBD a part of my wellness routine and feel better every day.

you. This is new for many doctors as well; I spoke to many who, like you, are generally curious and starting to gather their information. You may have to do a bit of searching to find a doctor who specializes in medical cannabis. I suggest you do three things:

1. Ask your own doctor. This might seem like a strange place to start—especially if you know that your doctor is not knowledgeable. But letting them know of your intention to try cannabis as part of your overall health plan is a crucial step.

2. Ask your friends and relatives. I was surprised at how many people I knew who had suggestions, recommendations, and stories. Not only was their information helpful, it once again showed me that I was in good company.

3. Turn to the web. Leafly.com and weedmaps.com provide information on doctors in your area.

How Do I Find and Visit a Dispensary?

First, know your state laws. Secondly, if you are in a state that allows medical marijuana, you will want to get a medical card for legal protection. Besides keeping everything on the up and up, medical marijuana is almost always less expensive than its recreational brethren. Sometimes it is more potent to allow for full medical benefits as well. If you are fortunate enough to live in a state where you can lawfully visit a dispensary, you should seize this educational opportunity. You may even find a friendly dispensary who has special hours and programs for beginners. Before visiting a marijuana dispensary, you should talk to your friends and doctor to see if they recommend a particular store. In addition, you'll want to visit a couple Web sites. Again, leafly.com and weedmaps.com are both highly rated and very user friendly. You can also usually go to a particular dispensary's Web site to read about them as well. When I get to a new place, I like to find someone to go with me for support, advice, safety, and frankly because it is just more fun.

Usually, there is a waiting room. Make sure you bring ID and your medical card if you have one. After your credentials are checked, you will enter the dispensary where—depending on the laws of your state—there may be two separate areas: one for recreational enthusiasts and one for medical patients. Sometimes certain products (such as edibles or medical oils) will only be available to medical patients. Medical patients often pay less for cannabis as well. And be sure

Questions to Ask Your Doctor

- Am I a good candidate for my condition to be treated with cannabis?

- If so, what method of cannabis consumption would you recommend?

- What dose should I start with and use during my course of treatment?

- Is there a particular brand of cannabis product that I should look for?

- Is the cannabis product I use going to get me high?

- What are the side effects of cannabis?

- Does cannabis interact with other medications?

- How long do the effects of cannabis last?

- Can I have a drink/glass of wine with cannabis?

- Am I eligible for a medical cannabis card?

- How will medical cannabis affect my daily routine?

- How do I stay safe while utilizing medical cannabis?

- Will I be able to utilize medical cannabis as a parent?

- What health care costs come along with medical cannabis?

- Are there activities I should avoid while utilizing medical cannabis?

- Can you refer me to other reliable sources for information on medical cannabis?

some questions about what you are looking for. Think of them as your personal concierge. They are more than happy to guide you through how to think about your purchase. Feel free to ask them if they have tried a particular product or how other customers have responded. Ask about their best sellers and why. Find out what strains and products they recommend for your style. And of course, ask them about the dosing and the price.

When you have made your purchase, you proceed to a register and make the transaction. Your products are given to you in child-resistant containers according to the laws of the state. And that's it. You just bought marijuana legally.

You'll have to do your research, but some states allow the convenience of delivery services. Common sense should rule your actions here. Try to get a referral before using a service, meet the delivery person in public, and bring a buddy. Also, check to see if there is a delivery fee or if there is a minimum order amount. If you are home bound, see if a friend can pick up your delivery for you in a public place.

It may be useful to look at the issues states have faced as they implement their medical cannabis programs to get a sense of what you may

to bring cash, as most dispensaries only take cash.

Once in your area, a dispensary employee called a budmaster or budtender greets you. They will ask you

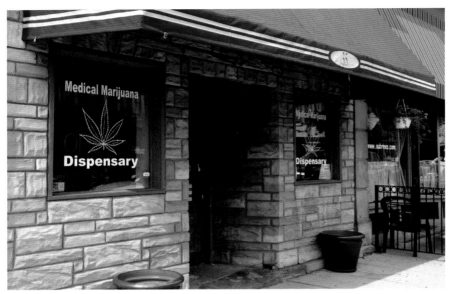

Welcome to the dispensary. Dispensaries vary widely in look and feel, but they are usually friendly settings that are now legitimate and regulated places of business.

expect in your state. Be aware that even the best-run medical cannabis programs still ask patients to face several hurdles. According to the ASA (Americans for Safe Access, which is a patient advocacy group) the top 10 best-run medical cannabis states are Illinois, Michigan, California, Oregon, Maine, New Mexico, Nevada, Montana, Ohio, and New Hampshire. The 10 worst-run programs—plus those states that have no medical cannabis program at all (six states in total including Idaho and Nebraska)—are Wisconsin, Tennessee, Missouri, Utah, Wyoming, Iowa, North Carolina, South Carolina, Alabama, and Mississippi.

The ASA used five factors to determine how effective states' programs are. Those factors are Patient Rights (including legal protection), Access to Medicine, Ease of Navigation, Functionality, and Consumer Safety. And bonus points were awarded to states who made improvements year over year. When we look at Illinois, which was the highest rated state, hurdles include the high cost of medicine and the limited number of dispensaries. In addition, patients must pass a background check and be fingerprinted. For patients who are home bound, they cannot order home delivery and cannot grow their own plants. In

Washington state, which is regarded as one of the most progressive states, the state has recently combined recreational and medical cannabis stores into a single storefront. This means that medical patients will be waiting in line with recreational customers, there is no state reciprocity, but patients can home grow. So again, every state has hurdles and you'll need to do research to find out the limitations you'll face (Americans for Safe Access 2018).

How Should I Store Cannabis? How Long Is It Potent?

The enemies of cannabis flower are heat, light, and mold, much like these elements affect everyday food products, such as cheese, bread, and berries. A simple and, honestly, the

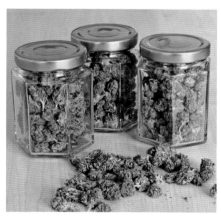

Storing cannabis. The best way to store cannabis is to put it in a sealed glass jar at or slightly below room temperature.

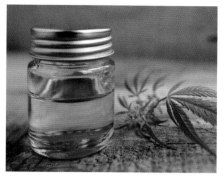

Careful storage pays off. Storing your infused oil in a cool, dark place maintains its potency and delicious, unique flavor.

best way to store weed is to put it in an airtight glass jar and keep it in a dark, room temperature, or cool place. Your refrigerator or freezer will degrade the buds, so don't ever put them in there. Plastic bags and plastic containers also detract from the potency of the cannabis because of static electricity and resin is attracted to the plastic. So, don't store your bud in plastic for any length of time. No matter how you store it, you should clearly label any cannabis flower that you have.

Infused oils and butters should be stored as you do normal olive oil, butter, and coconut oil—that is, store them in a dark, cool place. And you can store them in the refrigerator as well. The three main watchwords are cool, dark, and sealed. You can refrigerate your infused butter and it will last for several weeks. If you think you

Why Don't We Know More About the Benefits of Medical Cannabis?

While there is very interesting research coming from Israel, three agencies in the U.S. are severely hampering efforts to understand the therapeutic effects of cannabis, namely the National Institute on Drug Abuse (NIDA), the Drug Enforcement Agency (DEA), and the Food and Drug Administration (FDA). While U.S. university research has led the world to solve some of the most complex medical problems, approved cannabis research—complete with a growing operation—is off limits to nearly everyone. The University of Mississippi is the U.S.'s only approved grower. But even the University of Mississippi is hamstrung by a complex and confusing bureaucracy designed specifically to thwart research. If a scientist wants to conduct a study using cannabis, she starts by applying to NIDA. This is the first barrier. NIDA almost never gives permission, often citing the fact that cannabis is a Schedule I substance, which by definition means it has no medical benefits, so why would they let a doctor conduct research on this dangerous substance? But, that is only one of three approvals that the scientist must obtain. Next, they must move through the DEA. Again, because cannabis is still categorized as a Schedule I drug, the DEA barrier is obvious. Here is another place where the Schedule I designation causes a whole new set of (unforeseen) problems. And finally, the scientist (if she has the stomach, grit, and resources to devote to this) must get approval from the FDA. Only then can research start. But this red tape nightmare doesn't just hamper original research. Peer review and replication of results is what ultimately proves (or disproves) any research. If other universities can't grow cannabis or can't get approval, they can't replicate the studies or contribute to the collective understanding. And the cycle continues.

While there is much to be done, there are a couple of bright spots. There is a researcher in the U.S., George Kunos, who is a Principal Investigator (researcher) at the National Institute of Health; he is currently conducting research on the ECS system and had the following to say: "[the] endocannabinoid system...may have therapeutic potential in almost all diseases affecting humans, including obesity/metabolic syndrome, diabetes...neurodegenerative, inflammatory, cardiovascular, liver, gastrointestinal, skin diseases, pain, psychiatric disorders, cachexia, cancer, chemotherapy-induced nausea and vomiting, among many others" (Pacher and Kunos 2013, 1918-43).

Additionally, tenacious researcher Dr. Sue Sisley has recently been able to launch a study on the effects of CBD on PTSD. Her conviction cost her a teaching position at the University of Arizona, which did not want their brand associated with cannabis. But Dr. Sisley persisted and secured funding from the state of Colorado for her study; many veterans are anxious to hear the results. She has also applied to grow cannabis for medical studies because she was concerned about the lack of quality and variety of strains that the University of Mississippi was providing.

Profile

CONNECTING AND EDUCATING

ANTHONY DITTMANN, *Co-Founder of Cannabis Grand Cru,*
a Cannabis Events Company

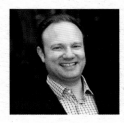

I entered the cannabis industry via a non-traditional route. Then again, there is little traditional about cannabis.

I grew up around cannabis (my family had plants in the backyard—even though we lived next door to a cop!), and of course I participated in it when I was younger. I am no longer an avid consumer; quite the contrary (however, I do wish it was my vice, as it is a much healthier vice than anything else out there). But that is also why I am such an advocate—not only for the love of the culture, but also to battle the hypocrisy and lobbying that occurs amongst the other much more detrimental drugs, big pharma and alcohol included. So many people just believe things, simply because they are told (and when we started our efforts, it was mind blowing to see how many people still believed in "reefer madness"). So my business partner and great friend Hezekiah and I decided to create an event called Cannabis Grand Cru (in Aspen, Seattle, and Portland). Our regular careers had us producing major televised events around the world for decades, and we found a void for professionals in any industry (you name it, banking, hotels, etc.) to join together and celebrate cannabis. We discovered such a tremendous community in cannabis. We found great people with a great cause, unsoiled by major corporations. A circle of smart, hardworking people who loved what they were doing, how they were doing it, and the end product. What is better than that?!

DID YOU KNOW?

Carl Sagan, the astronomer, astrophysicist, and Pulitzer author of *Cosmos*, wrote an essay in 1969 under the pen name Mr. X promoting the benefits and advocating for the legality of marijuana?

need longer shelf-life, consider freezing your butter. We find it handy to portion the butter into silicon ice cube trays and to make your dosage target 10 milligrams per butter cube. That way, if you want infused French Toast for breakfast one day, you can take out an infused butter cube, wait until it is at room temperature, and then spread the happiness. Infused butter

Profile

HOW I BECAME A FEDERAL MEDICAL CANNABIS PATIENT

And Why the Federal Government Has Not Wanted to Study My Protocol

IRVIN ROSENFELD, *Medical Cannabis Advocate, Stockbroker, and Survivor*

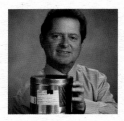

I am one of two remaining medical marijuana patients who successfully sued to get the U.S. government to send me cannabis; I receive 300 joints about every 25 days to help with the debilitating pain from a rare bone disorder. Still, the government does not want to research my long-term medical use.

I discovered the medical benefits of cannabis in the fall of 1971 and started learning about the federal prohibition against a plant that has been around for thousands of years. I also learned about the only legal grow in the U.S. that was started in 1968 on the campus of the University of Mississippi.

I started taking on the federal government in the fall of 1972. First, I had to get the Food and Drug Administration to approve my study on how cannabis enhanced the effects of Dilaudid (synthetic morphine). After that, we would have to contact the Drug Enforcement Agency to get their approval of the legality of my doctor and myself. Only then would the National Institute of Drug Abuse, with the approval of the other two agencies, ship out

the Schedule I Experimental New Drug to my doctor. Remember, this was 1972.

Needless to say, the powers that be had no intentions of helping anyone but the lobbyists who represented big pharmaceuticals. My doctor and I were not surprised by the lack of help from FDA. I kept the pressure on as best as I could.

In 1976, Robert Randall was arrested in Washington D.C. for growing a small amount of cannabis for his glaucoma. He went to court claiming medical necessity and was found not guilty. He had applied to the FDA to get cannabis from the government farm for his glaucoma, and having won in court, was granted access, at least for a little while (that's another story).

I met Robert in 1978 and, with his help, turned my medical study to the program he was now under called a "Compassionate Care Investigational New Drug Protocol." We reapplied to no avail. With the help of my Congressman, the Virginia State Police, and the state's Crime Commission, we doubled our efforts with the FDA. Still to no avail.

In early fall of 1979, I was lucky enough to get the University of Virginia Law School (UVA) to take up my cause. The FDA stonewalled UVA until the spring of 1982, when UVA threatened to sue the FDA in federal court. Finally, the leadership at the FDA gave in and held hearings for me in their headquarters in Rockville, Maryland, where I would have 15 minutes to convince a panel of 19 doctors that my project was valid.

I won those hearings and on November 20, 1982, I became the second person in the U.S. with a prescription for cannabis. The program increased to 13 patients before President George Bush senior shut the program down, "grandfathering" the 13 of us in. Today, there are only two of us left under the federal program.

Since 1937, the pharmaceutical, oil, paper, prisons, and other interested parties have been putting out false reports so they can keep control and continue making money. This is why they have never used any of my 70+ medical reports that have been submitted by my doctors for over 35 years.

This is why we need to continue to educate everyone about the wonderful medical aspects of this needed plant. Books like this one are very important.

For those who want to read my entire story, see *My Medicine: How I Convinced the U.S. Government to Provide My Marijuana and Helped Launch a National Movement* on Kindle, or for a signed copy see mymedicineconsulting.com.

in your freezer will last for about six months. When storing infused oil, treat it like a high-quality olive oil and keep it in a dark, cool place. When stored in this manner, your infused oil will retain its potency and can last for months.

The problem with mold

Mold is all around us. If you take a walk in the park, you are ingesting some mold. And for healthy adults, this is not an issue. But when it comes to marijuana, mold is a problem. Molds and mildews can release harmful, toxic chemicals called mycotoxins. Mycotoxins can affect your health in a variety of ways, including inducing lung infections and allergic reactions. If you consume moldy weed, you may experience a nagging cough, nose bleeds, chest pain, dizziness, fever, a feeling of being uncoordinated, and general overall fatigue.

Mold on cannabis looks like a white/grey spider web. If you see this, examine your flower more closely with a magnifying glass or a black light. If you find distinctive green spots, you likely have mold. If your product is moldy, don't smoke it, don't make edibles with it, and don't consume it in any other way. Sorry, you'll have to get rid of it.

Chapter 4

PERSONAL & RESPONSIBLE CONSUMPTION

There are many ways to consume cannabis. We will cover smoking and vaping, of course, but we will also explore using topical products, chewing infused gum, swallowing drops/tinctures, examining the world of edibles and infused drinks, and even consumption by suppository. Finally, we will mention a few "Advanced Methods," and then we'll end with a special discussion of CBD consumption. Remember, CBD on its own won't get you high, and is often used solely for health reasons.

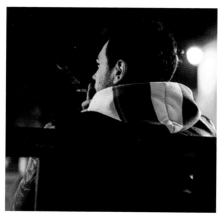

Burn one down. Smoking cannabis remains the most popular form of consumption, but vaping, edibles, and topicals are gaining in popularity.

Finding the "Right" Strain for You

On pages 47 and 48, we gave you a list of popular strains from the broad cannabis categories sativa, indica, hybrid, and strains high in CBD. These lists should serve as a good place to start. When you walk into a dispensary—especially for the first time—you will have your trusty lists to help guide your choices.

The "right" strain for you—and the method you use for consuming cannabis—completely depends on the type of experience you are looking for. Do you want something that will help you be more creative? Are you simply trying to relax at the end of the day? Are you searching for a strain that will help you handle your pain? Are you hoping to mitigate your anxiety? Do you enjoy getting high? Are you solely interested in using a form of CBD—which will not get you high? Is there a method of consumption that you prefer? Do you want to imbibe during the day? These questions will lead you to strains and products that may work for you.

When searching for different strains, you will find that a couple Web sites, namely leafly.com, cannasos.com, and cannabist.co (which is the official blog/cannabis Web site for the *Denver Post)*, include a wealth of information and several ways to search for strains. For example, on the cannasos.com site you can search by medical condition, by CBD, by THC, and by desired effect. Leafly.com is easy to navigate and provides a great depth of information, such as the usual THC and CBD potency of typical strains. This helps guide your choices if you are looking for a comfortable range of potency. Another plus that leafly.com offers is a peer review section where you can see how particular strains were described and rated by the cannabis community. Of course, the best and simplest thing you should do if you are a medical marijuana patient is to ask your doctor for a list of strains to start with. Conversely, if you are a recreation enthusiast, your best starting point is probably a knowledgeable friend. Also, as noted, if you go to a dispensary, feel free to ask the budtender/budmaster questions until you are comfortable.

Keeping a Journal

Keeping a cannabis journal is a very good idea, especially if you are just starting your cannabis journey. As a friend of mine pointed out, she wished someone had told her to keep notes about the different cannabis products she has tried from the beginning. She likened it to a wine journal and said that early on she would have a great bottle of wine and then promptly forget what the vintage and year was. Well, we want to make sure that doesn't happen to you with cannabis. So, we are encouraging you to keep a cannabis journal. Here are the basic topics you should cover and hey, it's your journal, so you should add what you want.

A cannabis journal is a small booklet that helps you keep track of how, when, and why you used a particular cannabis product and what the results were. If you are diligent about keeping a journal, you will be well on your way to becoming a responsible and knowledgeable cannabis user. A cannabis journal, then, helps you keep track of the following information:

- The strain, the quantity, the cost, and date purchased
- The name of the dispensary where product was purchased
- The potency of THC and/or CBD per serving; what is the serving size (that is, how much are you taking)?
- What product was consumed
- How it was consumed (that is, was it smoked, vaped, eaten as a gummy, etc.)
- What effects you observed and when they occurred. Possible observed effects may be euphoria, increased creativity, extra energy or lack of energy, increased focus or lack of focus, a feeling of relaxation (note whether it's mainly your body or mind, or both), different levels of pain relief, hunger, dry mouth, reduced (or increased) anxiety,

- level of sleepiness, and other noted effects
- Shortly after you finish feeling the effects, write a summary of how you feel
- How you felt one hour and two hours after consumption, and how you felt the next day
- In the back of your journal, you may want to write a master list of your favorite strains and other products after you've tested enough products

When you do this several times, you will begin to figure out what works for you, how you like to consume cannabis, and what effects you can expect. Be sure to start slowly and always use the lowest dose that works for you—no need to waste cannabis or to build up such a tolerance that you need more and more cannabis or stronger cannabis. A cannabis journal is available at OurCommunityHarvest. com or you can create your own.

Note that cannabis has become much more potent in recent years. If your recollection of cannabis was product you consumed in high school, you will be surprised. If you are just starting out, you should try low poten-cy strains. Low potency would be in the 0 to 10% THC range; the midrange is about 10 to 15% THC; and anything over 15% THC is pretty potent. You

will find that there may be some CBD present as well. For some people, this will provide pain relief, and when combined with some THC, will be a very pleasant experience.

Cannabis and the Use of Alcohol and Tobacco

One notable side effect is some can-nabis users find using cannabis helps cut down on alcohol consumption. In a January 2018 article in *Forbes* mag-azine, a 10-year study spearheaded by the University of Connecticut looked at alcohol sales data in states that allow medical cannabis. They found that the use of alcohol was down by 15%. The researchers concluded that cannabis and alcohol function as strong substitutes for each other because they share a similar audience. Anecdotally, I have heard a good number of cannabis users admit that they have consciously cut down or eliminated their use of alcohol in favor of cannabis, primarily due to health concerns (Pellechia 2018).

Some users of both tobacco and cannabis use their cannabis vapes to help them cut down on cigarette smoking. It may be the habitual nature of having something to smoke, or replacing the effects of cigarettes with the effects of cannabis, but vape pens are replacing some cigarettes—hopefully this is a good trend. A research team led by C. Hindocha had this to say in the *Journal of Addiction:* "there could be reason to be optimistic about the potential of vaporizers. If vaporizers can reduce cannabis and tobacco co-administration, the outcome could be a reduction of tobacco use/dependence among cannabis users and a resultant reduction in harms associated with cannabis. Indeed, if vaping cannabis becomes commonplace in the future, the next generation of cannabis users might never be exposed to nicotine or tobacco in the first place" (Hindocha, Freeman, Winstock, Lynskey 2016).

A Note on CBD Consumption

A 2013 study published in the *British Journal of Clinical Pharmacology* found CBD helpful in reducing nausea, suppressing seizures, combatting psychotic disorders, battling inflammation, and more. Before starting to use CBD products, check with your doctor and make sure to tell them what medications you are already taking.

Weigh your consumption options: you can find a flower strain that is high in CBD and low in THC and smoke it or vape it. You can use a topical product, like a CBD lotion or salve, and put it on affected areas. You could take liquid drops or chew CBD gum. You could try commercially available edibles, infused coffee, tea, or other beverages, or perhaps try a suppository. Or you could learn to cook with it once you have properly dosed CBD oil or butter. We'll cover the creation of edibles in chapter 6.

Methods of Consumption

In terms of consumption, the methods covered here apply to the ingestion of both THC and CBD products—and products that contain both elements.

Smoking

Some of us remember starting our relationship with cannabis by smoking a joint, or a rolled marijuana cigarette, with a bunch of friends. Or you may have passed around a pipe or a bong. Some of you may have even tried a blunt, which is a cigar "wrapper" (the outside tobacco leaf of a small cigar) filled with cannabis and rolled; the blunt stays lit and burns slowly. (In the U.S., a cannabis cigarette is called a joint, but in Europe, a traditional joint is called a blunt; make sure to clarify what you are consuming). You may have also heard the word spliff; this is a combination of tobacco and cannabis that is rolled together and smoked. The high is intensified because of the tobacco. There are also products called "One Hitters" that are about the size of a deck of cards; usually a little wooden box with two chambers. The first, slightly larger chamber holds a bit of cannabis and the second chamber holds a hollow metal tube that you fill by pushing down into the cannabis chamber and then you smoke. If you've seen the show *Entourage*, the guys often carry a one hitter on the golf course and when out in public.

There are even more creative smoking methods, like making a pipe out of an apple or a soda can. If you look online, you will see these and other smile-inducing creative smoking methods. All of these devices—joints, blunts, pipes, bongs, and one hitters—are very common ways of smoking marijuana. Generally, you take a bud, grind it, cut it, or tear it apart in small pieces, and then roll a joint or put it in the device and heat it without burning it (if possible).

Smoking yields quick relief and a way to easily control dosing and consumption; the medicine will be delivered quickly, within about 5 minutes. The smoke goes into the lungs and then is rapidly disbursed into the bloodstream. When you smoke cannabis, purists recommend that you hold the smoke in for 3 or 4 seconds, which

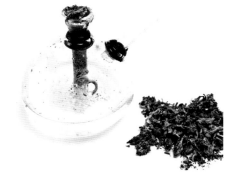

Keep it simple. Or not. The most commonly known and perhaps oldest method of consumption is through smoking, which can be done in a variety of ways.

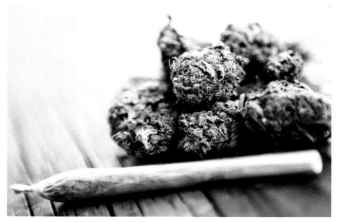

starts the high. You should try not to touch or handle the bud too much, or the resin will stick to your fingers and you'll lose some potency. And when you light your pipe, try to keep the flame right above the cannabis so you heat it enough to activate its potency, but not enough to light the bud on fire. If your bud is on fire, put it out right away and do not put the flame so far into the pipe next time. Some cannabis purists will even tell you that you shouldn't use a lighter because the butane will affect the taste of your bud, and that you should use a match instead. Honestly, most of us can't tell the difference and it doesn't seem to harm the experience. Here is an interesting fact to keep in mind—the potency of a joint increases as the joint gets smaller. So, if you smoke half a joint, you only get about 25% of the potency of the whole joint; by the time you get to the roach (the little, roughly last inch of the joint), you are smoking the most potent part of the joint.

A Bit More Information About Blunts and Spliffs. Blunts and spliffs are similar to joints, but have increased effects because they are rolled with tobacco. Blunts are cigar wrappers that have been filled with cannabis and smoked; nicotine is ingested from the wrapper. Spliffs are joints that are filled with a combination of tobacco and cannabis. If you are not already a cigarette or tobacco smoker, it is unlikely that blunts and spliffs will appeal to you, and you may not want to face the health risks associated with smoking tobacco.

In terms of absorption, smoking marijuana is one of the fastest ways to feel a high, and generally you will note effects in about 5 minutes. The smoke enters your lungs and then is distributed in the bloodstream, which happens relatively quickly. And depending on the strain and your physical makeup, you can expect to be high for about 1 to 3 hours. If your strain has an element of THC, you may feel effects in your head as well as your body.

Newcomers to smoking cannabis may have a picture of Cheech and Chong, Harold and Kumar, or the characters from *Dazed and Confused.* You know, the guys who kept smoking well after they were stoned. But responsible consumption starts with going low and slow. As a new user, you should smoke just a pinch—taking a puff or two—and then wait and see how you feel. Yes, I know as Tom Petty said that "waiting is the hardest part," and you may be tempted to smoke as much cannabis as you can while you are waiting for the effects to start. But by doing this you are probably smoking too much, and you aren't figuring how much (really how little) cannabis you need to imbibe to get the effect you want. If you overconsume, you are also building up your tolerance, which may lead to increased use and wanting more potent product. So be smart, learn how your body reacts, and deliberately enjoy the journey.

Vaping

One alternative to smoking is vaping, which provides relief in about 15 minutes. Vaping heats the cannabis to the point before combustion (about 340°), and because it doesn't combust, it is reportedly healthier than smoking because it does not release the toxins that smoking does. Vaping is more like ingesting infused steam and is discreet and portable. Like smoking, hold in the vapor for a few seconds, exhale, take note of your condition after about 15 minutes, and continue in this manner until you are comfortable. Smoking and vaping are some of the fastest ways to get relief. As with smoking, the vapor enters the lungs and then is moved into the bloodstream.

Vaping has become hugely popular because it is discreet, portable, and probably healthier than smoking a joint, pipe, or bong. Vaping is done with a vape pen, which is a small, battery-operated handheld inhaler, or a larger desktop unit like the Volcano; they work with cannabis bud or cannabis concentrate, liquid drops that come in a cartridge.

Vape Pens. Vape pens can also hold multiple doses at a time, which is convenient. Another popular vape product is the disposable

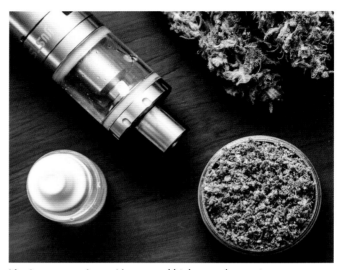

Next-era vaporizers. Newer and higher-end vaporizers are efficient and effective ways to consume cannabis in a way that is thought to be safer than smoking.

vape pen, with a single pen often giving hundreds of little doses. One advantage of vape pens is that you can take a single puff, see how you feel in about 5 to 15 minutes, and if more is needed, a second puff or even more can be inhaled. Vape pens work with both CBD and THC oil or a combination. Finally, vape pens are portable and discreet. While traditional smoking methods are still the most popular, some surmise that "vapes" will become the most popular ingestion method soon.

If you are a parent, one thing to watch out for is a trend for underage students to vape with flavored juices (which may or may not contain nicotine) and other liquids, and may occa-

Profile

BREAKING THE GRASS CEILING

ASHLEY PICILLO, *Founder of Point Seven Group and Author Focusing on Women in the Cannabis Industry*

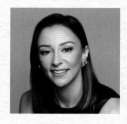

I was 100% a D.A.R.E. kid. While my parents are extremely liberal on most fronts, they were staunchly opposed to "drugs." Because I was the oldest kid—and a female—my parents watched me like a hawk. I was a classic over-achiever by all accounts and, by way of my upbringing, saw marijuana as something that could only derail me from my plans. While I certainly became more open-minded during college, I refrained from consuming. In the fall of 2013, a strange series of events unfolded and the idea of moving to Colorado in advance of legalization was presented to me. I was slated to start an operations job in New York, but had a few months to kill and had always wanted to spend time in Colorado, so I packed up a suitcase and hit the road.

I quickly found myself immersed in this "industry," and realized a few things: 1) Cannabis is not a drug. It is a plant and a medicine; and 2) As someone who thoroughly enjoys building and designing systems, I realized that I had an incredible opportunity to help build something that had never been built before.

I spent the next two years intimately involved in the Colorado market heading up operations for a vertically integrated facility where I had my hands in just about everything from dispensing to post-harvest to product development, extraction, and distribution. It was the steepest, most rewarding learning curve of my life and, because of this experience, I was equipped with almost every tool I needed to take this knowledge on the road (almost representing the incredible team I did not yet have). In 2016, I launched Point Seven Group to support companies around the country in procuring licenses to grow, dispense, or process. Since then, my entirely (badass) women-run team has grown to support a wide range of services for the industry including facility design, equipment sourcing, licensing, SOP development, marketing, branding, and more.

In 2017, I authored *Breaking the Grass Ceiling* with a lifelong friend-turned-colleague of mine, Lauren Devine, which connected me with 21 pioneering cannabis women. I wanted to create this biographical collection to educate female newcomers in the industry, while showcasing the incredible professionals working in cannabis. It has been the greatest adventure of my life and I look forward to spending the foreseeable future advocating for patients and policy reform, while working to shift the mindsets of people thinking the way I was only a few years ago.

sionally try to vape cannabis. If they are vaping cannabis, it is difficult to detect as vapes only give off a bit of tell-tale smell. But you should be able to notice subtle changes in behavior or detect red eyes and possibly more deliberate movement on the part of your child. Remind your children that their brains continue growing and developing well into their 20s, so it's recommended that they do not use cannabis until they are 25 years old (DEA "Drugs of Abuse - Marijuana").

Desktop Vaping Machines. Desktop machines like the popular Volcano collect vape "smoke" in a plastic balloon; the user inhales from the balloon. Volcanoes are relatively expensive machines, but use a minimal amount of cannabis; an exact temperature can be selected and dosage can be easily controlled.

Tincture or Liquid Drops

A tincture is liquid that is infused with active cannabis ingredients. It is often made with high-proof alcohol that evaporates and you are left with potent drops that work well in an eye dropper. If you put a dropperful under your tongue and wait for about 30 seconds before swallowing, you will feel the effects in about 15 minutes. The drops are absorbed sublingually,

which is a relatively effective way to take medicine and doesn't require the user to swallow a pill. When cannabis was widely used as medicine in the last half of the 19th century, it was offered as drops or tinctures. So, in some ways, we are coming full circle.

A dramatic demonstration of the power of tinctures was outlined on page 56 when we discussed the little girl named Charlotte who had repetitive epileptic episodes. A special infused tincture made out of a new cannabis strain, now called Charlotte's Web, helped to radically limit her seizures. This is just one example of how a medical need for CBD led to the creation of a new strain and a popular CBD product. And in part because of the advocacy of parents of epileptic children, even some traditionally conservative states like Utah and Oklahoma now allow CBD drops as a medical option for epilepsy.

One of the reasons that drops are popular is because they are discreet, quick acting, and easy to use and dose. Most users are encouraged to take drops a couple of times a day rather than merely once a day at their preferred dose. If you are going to try drops—as with any cannabis product— remember that we suggest that you speak to a physician who specializes in cannabis.

Pets and Cannabis

Have you heard that pet owners are giving their pets cannabis for various ailments and issues such as separation anxiety, pain, and sleeplessness? It is not yet legal for vets to prescribe cannabis. They can provide education, but they are not supposed to dispense medical advice/recommendations. As with humans, it appears that dogs and cats can have adverse reactions to THC, so most pet owners stick with solely CBD products. There are several lines of CBD-infused dog treats available on the market. We order Pure Hemp Collective 25 mg CBD pet treats as they have no THC. Friends of ours use it to help their rescued greyhound ease pain from a racing injury. Another option outside of pet treats are drops. Drops, as you recall, work faster, but it may be easier to give your pet a treat. If you do decide to use cannabis for your pet, make sure to monitor for overconsumption—primarily of THC—look for symptoms such as diarrhea, vomiting, and balance issues.

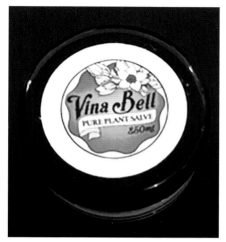

It couldn't get easier. Applied just as any body lotion would be, salves are simple to use. That said, determining the proper dosage often requires a process of trial and error.

Topical Cannabis

Let's not forget topical products, which are absorbed through our largest organ, the skin. Topical products include lotions, salves, pain sprays, and transdermal patches and are applied directly to affected areas such as sore knees; the topical then goes to work fighting inflammation where it was applied. Cannabis topicals are a relatively new area of cannabis consumption that are heavily or solely composed with CBD. By and large, even if the topical contains THC, the user will not get high. The exception is that some powerful transdermal patches may induce a high.

If you have aches, pains, and inflammation, topicals such as lotions, balms, salves, liquid pain spray, and transdermal patches may provide relief. So instead of reaching for a commercial analgesic for your arthritis or sports injury, for example, check with your doctor and you may be directed to topical cannabis.

When using topical cannabis products, like any cannabis product, start with a low dose and see how your body responds (are you noting a pattern here?). Salves, which are as simple to apply as commercial lotion, should be rubbed into the affected area; then monitor yourself throughout the day. Because absorption into the skin is not the most efficient delivery method, it will most likely take some personal experimentation to find out how much topical product to use. And do not apply topicals to sensitive areas.

Suppositories

Although it may make you a bit uncomfortable to think about using a cannabis-infused suppository, you may want to consider using this method for a couple of reasons. First, you may not be able to take a pill, or you might have nausea that limits your ingestion of edibles, and you might also not want to try other methods like smoking or vaping. Second, suppositories provide much quicker relief than edibles do. Suppositories generally start to work in about 15 minutes or less and they deliver an efficient amount of medicine to the body quickly.

Suppositories are also very easy to use. Consult your doctor and start with a conservative dose. When using the suppository, it is as simple as placing the suppository in your rectum past the sphincter (which means the suppository should go in about an inch and a half to two inches). After insertion, remain calm and comfort-

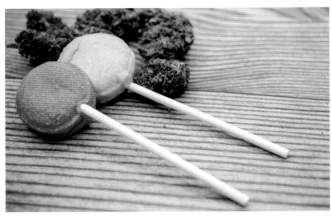

Edibles come in all forms. Edibles range from lollipops to baked breads and take effect more slowly than smoking or vaporizing.

able, and relief will start in about 10 to 15 minutes.

There are also suppositories for vaginal use. Vaginal suppositories have been found to provide fast relief from cramps and pelvic discomfort for women suffering from period- and pelvic-related pain. They can also be used to enhance sex; some users swear by a related product, namely "weed lube." Cannabis or weed lube provides moisture, relieves pain, and relaxes the user—all of which helps to explain its new-found popularity.

Edibles/Medibles

Many people associate cannabis with smoking, but one of the fastest growing modes of consumption is via edibles (or, because they are infused with cannabis, they are sometimes

Profile

BACK DOOR MEDICINE

PAULA-NOEL MACFIE, PH.D

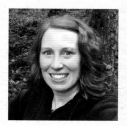

I am a philosopher, educator, public speaker, author, junior high sports coach, and Girl Scout Troop Leader. I started a business called Back Door Medicine LLC, whose primary mission is to publish, research, and educate decolonizing research methodologies.

I am also a medical patient with a doctoral research background, navigating my own health challenges and serving those around me with my developing research methods and resources. I was diagnosed with clinical depression at age 16 and began using cannabis to self-medicate by age 17. I also had suffered from traumatic brain injury and sexual assault.

When I was 31 years old, I finished my doctoral degree after spending over six years with indigenous elders and healers from clans and tribes around the world. Within months of graduating, I was diagnosed with multiple sclerosis. Recently, I was also diagnosed with Aspberger's (high functioning) and ADHD. Within all of the health obstacles, I have managed to obtain an advanced degree and continue to develop research methods that not only help me with my own health, but others who are suffering.

I am independent from the recreational cannabis community. I provide suppository molds at a low cost to people who choose to make cannabis suppositories themselves. I educate people on the process I have used personally and am gathering testimonies of others who have done the same.

Back Door Medicine LLC's primary purpose is to provide research and education in the areas of whole food plant-based nutrition, chronic/terminal conditions, genealogy, indigenous science, recovery of indigenous mind, and decolonization. After experiencing an extremely unpleasant anal fissure, I was *desperate* after everything western homeopathic and alternative did not work.

I read about Tommy Chong healing his prostate cancer with cannabis suppositories. I didn't think twice. I ordered a $175 mold, went to my local dispensary, and purchased some organic extra-virgin coconut oil (I recommend cacao butter now). Over seven days of pain were eliminated in two days. I thought, "If this can help me, it must help other people with a variety of conditions." I wish I had known when my brother was alive and suffering from rectal and liver cancer. Because of this, when I had my first cannabis suppository tested, I named it Jeff's Wish.

I officially started a business in November 2015 to provide support, research, and education in various areas. Back Door Medicine LLC includes cannabis suppository education, mold accessibility at a fair and reasonable price, and decolonizing research methods.

referred to as medibles). In simplest terms, an edible is food or beverage that has been infused with cannabis. If you are thinking "pot brownie," you are thinking of the classic example of an edible.

We'll go into cooking with cannabis and serving edibles a little later in the book, but here are some general guidelines for you when it comes to edibles. First, the experience is entirely different from smoking marijuana. When you smoke cannabis, you normally feel the effects in approximately 5 minutes and the sensation may be largely cerebral. With edibles, whether you are big or small, male or female, a devoted or casual user, it could take anywhere from 30 minutes to 2 hours to feel the effects, and for many it is more of a body high; the edibles must travel through the stomach, liver, and intestines, which is why the effects take a while to kick in. A few factors that can slightly quicken the time that edibles take effect are if you have an empty stomach, have consumed alcohol, or have just eaten a sugary snack.

Because you just don't know how edibles will affect you until you try them, we recommend going low and slow—that is, start with a low dose, take your time, and don't add alcohol or other forms of marijuana, or your effects will be heightened—possibly to an uncomfortable level. Once the effects kick in they will last a long time, with some users reporting effects lasting 4 to 8 hours. Eating edibles at a slow pace and then sleeping peacefully is a favorite and achievable goal of edible fans.

It is ridiculously easy to overconsume edibles because their effects take so long to kick in and the temptation to have a second serving or a quick puff while you are "waiting" is hard to resist. To avoid this unpleasant possibility, we encourage you to make edibles a mindful, deliberate experience. So as far as dosing goes, be conservative. I might even start with a 2.5 milligram serving and see how it goes. And yes, there is a chance that you will not feel anything. This means that the next time you try edibles, you can try a 5 milligram dose and note how you feel. You'll find your right level as you increase your intake gradually. But again, above all, go low and slow when it comes to edibles. Remember, size doesn't seem to matter. Just because you might be bigger doesn't mean your body needs more.

Advanced Methods

Since this is an introductory book on cannabis, we aren't going to cover what I would call advanced methods of consumption. But you may hear people talking about shatter, wax, dabbing, hash oil, and smoking hash—all of which are designed for experienced and serious marijuana consumers—some of which can be potentially dangerous. Especially if you create these products yourself, as they often use butane or other solvents, you have to be careful. These products are all concentrated versions of cannabis, and if you consume them, you will find that they pack a punch. To compare: a strong joint can contain up to 30% THC, whereas a dab may have potency of up to 90%! Of course, if you are curious about any of these products or ingestion techniques, a little research on the Web will tell you all you want to know.

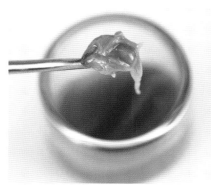

The cutting edge. Shatter, or wax, is a form of dabs, the catch-all term for highly potent marijuana concentrates that produce intense highs; definitively not for novices.

What Safety Issues Should I Be Aware Of?

There are a few issues you should keep in mind before beginning your cannabis consumption.

Dosing

The first thing is to understand dosing. Although it is reported widely that no one has died from cannabis and you cannot overdose on cannabis, like any medication, there are some cautions that should be respected. The first thing, naturally, is to ask your doctor. Here are some general rules to keep in mind while determining appropriate dosing for yourself:

- With your doctor, figure out how you want to consume your medicine— weigh the advantages and limitations of smoking, vaping, topicals, edibles and infused beverages, gum, tinctures, and suppositories.
- Start with a very low dose several times a day (new users sometimes start out with doses as low as 2.5 milligrams two to three times a day).
- Once you feel relief, continue to use your product of choice at the lowest effective level.
- If your dose is becoming less effective, slowly and carefully increase your consumption.

Child Safety

Each state has child safety regulations that you should know and respect. At a minimum, dispensaries sell cannabis products that you take home in child-safe containers. And once you get home, be sure that your product is clearly labeled and is stored in a safe place that is inaccessible to children. You should also keep your cannabis products away from pets. But know that some vets will recommend CBD for pets and there are specific products such as infused pet treats that are available for your furry friends (page 158).

Driving

It should go without saying, but do not consume cannabis and drive. You may feel like you are in control, but your reactions are slowed, and you could face some serious legal consequences. Let's keep the roads safe and not give cannabis opponents an excuse to curtail the progress we've made. Be aware that in many states if you have an accident and are subject to a drug test that you will test positive for cannabis long after you have used cannabis. In fact, if you are a daily user and stopped use for a month you may still test positive! This means that even though you would be sober at the time of an accident, you may still

be charged. So just don't consume and drive.

Mental Health

In reviewing some medical cannabis literature and looking at anecdotal cannabis stories, it appears that you should use caution if you or your family have a history of mental health issues. Specifically, if you or your family have a history of chronic depression, bipolar symptoms, or schizophrenia, cannabis—especially cannabis high in THC—should be used with caution and under the guidance of a physician as it may increase anxiety. Conversely, it may be the case that your doctor will recommend that you start with CBD, which has been found to combat anxiety.

Pulmonary Issues

Be aware that smoking cannabis increases your heart rate, so if you have pulmonary issues, again, tread lightly and carefully. In this case, other forms of consumption such as edibles, topicals, and suppositories would all be better choices than smoking. Vaping may be a bit safer as well.

What Do I Do If I Have an Uncomfortable High?

Unfortunately, it happens sometimes— you've gotten yourself too high. If this

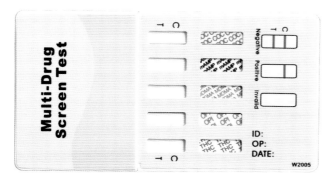

If you need to know. Curious about results on an upcoming drug test? An over-the-counter test kit can be a good first step to make sure you are clean.

happens, first, try to remain calm. And if you are with friends, let someone you trust know how you are feeling. Then, here are a few things you can try:

- You should hydrate, so drink a room-temperature glass of water.
- You can try to rest or sleep if you are in a place where that's okay.
- Some people respond well to going for a walk (accompanied, of course). Walking and talking can often distract your brain from focusing on the high.
- There is some evidence that if you smell or chew black peppercorns this will provide relief as well. Reportedly, this was a method that the singer Neil Young recommended.
- Finally, some folks respond well to ingesting some CBD to counteract the THC. If you can locate CBD drops or gum, these products can enter your system relatively quickly and may offer some relief.

- Once you've recovered—which may just mean you've had a solid night of sleep—reflect on what went wrong and make sure not to repeat your missteps.

What If I Might Have to Take a Drug Test?

It happens. You go for the job of your dreams and the drug test is part of their process. The best scenario is knowing you are going to be tested so you can stop your consumption immediately and for a while. If you are an occasional user, tests may detect marijuana in your system for 1 to 5 days. If you are a regular user, cannabis can stay in your system 1 to 3 weeks. If you use multiple times in a single day, it may take 4 to 6 weeks for your system to be clear. But it isn't all bad news here: For heavy users, if and when you resume use, you will feel effects more quickly and more profoundly. It's a bit like starting to use for the first time!

It is always helpful to flush out your system with water, so be sure to heavily hydrate for a couple days. If you are taking a urine test, do not use your first urine of the day. And do not use the beginning of your urine stream either, try to use urine that is about halfway in your stream later in the day. Beyond that, refer to norml.org, where they discuss various

METHODS OF CONSUMPTION AND EFFICIENCY

Method	Time for Effect	*Efficiency	Advantages/Drawbacks
Smoking (including joints, pipes and bongs)	Approximately 5 minutes	Good	Simple, quick acting/Loss of potency
Blunts	5 minutes	Good	Simple, quick acting/Tobacco ingestion, loss of potency
Spliffs	5 minutes	Good	Simple, quick acting/Tobacco ingestion, loss of potency
Vapes	15 minutes	Good	Discreet, portable, quick acting/Loss of potency
Tincture/Drops	15 minutes	Good	Easy to use and dose, quick acting/Some may have difficulty swallowing
Infused Gum	15 to 30 minutes	Good	No need to swallow, quick acting, precise dosing/Challenge for those who have trouble with chewing, dental, and jaw problems
Edibles/Medibles	30 minutes to 2 hours	Poor	Many choices/Hard to dose correctly, loses a lot of potency
Topicals	Difficult to calculate	Very Poor	Direct application, many products/Loses most potency
Suppositories	15 minutes	Excellent	Quick acting, retains most potency/Rectal or vaginal insertion
Nasal Spray	15 minutes	Good	Easy to use and dose/Uncomfortable for some
Transdermal Patches	15 minutes	Good	Enters body efficiently/Sensitive skin may limit use

*Efficiency refers to length of time required for the product to take effect, how much "medicine" is delivered, and how easily the body absorbs and uses it.

types of drug tests, which are most effective and more. It's a class in itself!

Other Issues

Even though medical cannabis is legal in most of the U.S., you may face some backlash regarding its use. Regular cannabis use may mean that your life insurance premiums increase. Some employers may conduct drug tests and refuse to recognize the benefits

DID YOU KNOW?

Reefer Madness, the 1936 film that became the propaganda beacon of the federal government's anti-marijuana campaign, was originally financed by a church group? After it was shot, it was purchased by a producer who added much of the campy, salacious content for distribution on the emerging exploitation film circuit.

of medical cannabis. But if you use synthetic THC (Marinol, also known as Dronabinol), in a drug test it will come up as negative. This will likely be a difficult decision for you and you'll have to weigh the benefits and risks associated with medical cannabis use. I wish you courage and wisdom.

Profile

SOLVING A CANNABIS SAFETY PROBLEM—WITH STYLE

SKIP STONE, *CEO of Stashlogix*

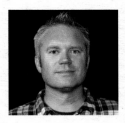

Hi, I'm Skip Stone, CEO of Stashlogix. Before Stashlogix, I was your average dad who was enjoying newly legal cannabis in Colorado. And I had a problem—with two young kids and a new puppy, I was worried they might get into my stash, especially my edible THC-infused gummy bears. Because I'm an engineer, I set out to solve the problem.

I prototyped a storage bag with an integrated lock. I also invented an odor control system and added organizational features for cannabis. I showed it to my friends and they all wanted one.

Realizing I was onto something, I applied to the first class of CanopyBoulder. Canopy-Boulder is the first start-up accelerator and business incubator specific to the cannabis industry. Getting accepted out of 120 applicants was the "ah-ha" moment I needed to get in at the ground-level of a budding new industry.

Since then, we've been creating a lifestyle storage brand that appeals to the "new can-nabis consumer": soccer moms, athletes, businessmen, and baby boomers. Our products can help them be discreet, stay organized, and keep others from accessing their stuff.

While the Canadian government is actively promoting and likely to be purchasing our products as a common-sense solution to keep kids safe from cannabis, in 2017 the U.S. government seized a shipment of our products in Customs, blocking us from importing. Most businesses in this industry have their share of war stories, but most very are passionate about the plant and want to help break the stigma—we're with them.

The biggest story that came out of Colorado in 2014 were all the kids that were sent to the ER due to accidental cannabis edibles consumption. While the problem was blown out of proportion by the media, it is one of the real fall-outs from legalization. I think our products solved that, at least to some extent. In addition to safety, we're helping people be discreet, because handling cannabis is tricky; it's messy, dirty, sticky, and smelly. We want to help people so they're not judged for choosing a healthier alternative to alcohol or a natural alternative to pharmaceuticals.

Chapter 5

MAKING YOUR OWN INFUSIONS FOR EDIBLES

An edible is simply food that is infused with cannabis. Most people think of the classic pot brownie as an edible, but today there are new cooking techniques and many edible choices. The creation of cannabis edibles has become big business in dispensaries, and there are also accomplished chefs who create gourmet meals. Popular edible products at dispensaries include chocolate, gummies, baked goods, ice cream, infused drinks from coffee to sodas, and all kinds of candy. And at home, edible cooks can create and infuse nearly any dish.

Here's a secret about making infused cannabis edibles: you simply infuse butter and oil, and then cook as you normally do. However, infusing oil or butter takes a bit more effort than crumbling up some bud in oil and adding it to a brownie mix. While it might take a bit more effort, you will be able to simply create and store enough infused oils and butters for much more than a tray of brownies! We will discuss a few different methods to infuse oil or butter, but regardless of method, it is important to know how much cannabis you have infused into your oil or butter. We'll talk about dosing as well.

Some of the most popular types of infusions are:

- Olive oil
- Butter
- Coconut oil
- Vegetable oil
- Ghee (clarified butter)
- Honey, walnut oil, avocado oil, or maple syrup

I love to cook and to entertain (see page 140). I have found that it is most helpful if you have a few infusions available to choose from as you cook. For versatile daytime use, infused olive oil is my go-to. I find that it works well as a drizzle for lunch, dinner, and dinner parties. When baking or making desserts, infused coconut oil usually gets the call. As a versatile ingredient that freezes well, infused butter is handy. So, if you keep all of these infusions available, you should be able to infuse nearly any cuisine.

The Basics of Infusing

While many of us may have experimented with infusing by trying to make the ever-popular pot brownies, we may have skipped a step or two. Fast forward to today and there are many cannabis chefs who have learned how to create infusions, calculate dosage, and even pair particular strains with certain cuisines and wines. Notably, these chefs often are happy to share their techniques and

List of Kitchen Items Needed for Cannabis Cooking

Here is a list of items that you should keep separate from your other cookware and use solely for cooking with cannabis:

- A sharp knife, paring size or larger
- Good strainer
- Mason jars of assorted sizes
- Measuring cups and measuring spoons
- Labels (or masking tape) and marker for labeling
- Scale
- Wooden spoon
- Silicone ice cube tray (for storing infused butter)
- Deep pan for simmering
- Cutting board
- Baking sheet for decarboxylating
- Cheesecloth

what they have learned by trial and error, which means that we now know the best steps to make infusions.

Simple Methods for Decarboxylating and Infusing

The first step in preparing your infusion is something called decarboxylation or slow roasting. Decarboxylating your cannabis is not hard, but it is a key step in creating infused meals.

This step activates the THC and/or CBD in your flower. Decarboxylation leads to maximum potency and helps the consumer to better measure and dose correctly. If you skip this step, you are wasting much of your product's potency. So, don't skip this step!

Decarboxylating can be done in a few ways: oven roasting, sous vide, or mason jar/water bath.

First, choose a cannabis strain that has the attributes you desire, such as high CBD or low THC. The THC and/or CBD potency of your cannabis should be verified by a dispensary or a testing device. You can then use a dosing calculator—such as the one available at OurCommunityHarvest.com/Calculator—to calculate potency of your infusion (see more on page 98).

One note about the decarboxylation process—you won't be able to mask what you are doing, unless you use the sous vide or mason jar techniques (described in chapter 5). The aroma is strong and smells just like you think it does! As soon as you start decarbing, your kitchen, possibly most of your house, and even a bit of your neighborhood will smell like weed. Some cannacooks cover their roasting pan/cookie sheet with a lid or foil, which lessens the smell a bit, but it is still there. Another way you can mitigate the smell is with good ventilation. Another trick is to make cinnamon rolls or a roasted garlic dish to mask the odor.

If you prefer to learn visually, The Cannabist Web site has a good infusion video: thecannabist.co/2013/12/27/kitchenweed/1244/

Always be sure to mark the potency of your infusion; note the strength of both a tablespoon and a teaspoon, since these are common cooking measurements (see page 98).

Store infused butter in the refrigerator or freezer, and your oil in a cool, dark place. If storing butter in the freezer, a silicone ice cube tray with 10 milligrams of infused butter in each cube works well.

Oven

The traditional way to decarb cannabis is in the oven or toaster oven.

1. Preheat the oven to 200°F.
2. To make 16 ounces of infused oil or butter, start with ¼ ounce (7 grams) of cannabis. Crumble, cut or tear the cannabis.
3. Spread the cannabis on a cookie sheet in a single layer.
4. Roast for 60 to 90 minutes, checking every 15 minutes or so to make sure it is roasting evenly. Cannabis should be dry, but not burnt.

5. Let decarbed cannabis cool to room temperature and then wrap in cheesecloth.
6. Using a saucepan, bring 16 ounces of oil or butter to a slow simmer. If using butter, add a cup of water; it will steam out during the steeping process, but will keep your butter at the right consistency.
7. Place the wrapped cannabis in the saucepan and simmer for 60 to 90 minutes; press cheesecloth about every 15 minutes with a spoon.
8. Let cool to room temperature. Strain oil/butter through a strainer lined with cheesecloth into a mason jar.
9. Mark your infusion with potency (see page 98) and strain.

Sous Vide

A sous vide is a simple device that uses water and a vacuum-sealed plastic bag to heat food to a precise temperature and keep it there. That means you can't really burn anything in a sous vide, and it produces no odor. Many high-end restaurants use this method to serve dishes such as salmon, steak, and chicken. Sous vide devices are not that expensive, and they are not bulky. Note that if you don't have a sous vide, you can use a slow cooker as long as it stays at a

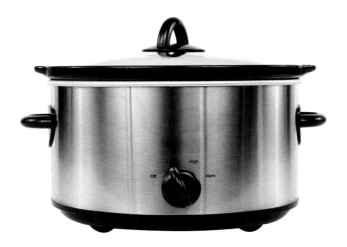

Keep it simple The equipment required for cooking with cannabis are no different than what is likely already in your kitchen.

consistent temperature. You may want to periodically check the temperature in your slow cooker with a thermometer. Also, sous vides have submersible racks that holds the cannabis in place under the water. With a slow cooker, make sure to weigh down your cannabis so it doesn't float.

1. Fill a pot or heat-proof container of appropriate size with water and set the sous vide device to 200°F.

2. To make 16 ounces of infused oil or butter, start with ¼ ounce (7 grams) of cannabis. Crumble, cut or tear the cannabis.

3. Fill your vacuum bag with the cannabis and seal it according to manufacturer directions.

4. Place the bag in the sous vide for about an hour.

5. Let decarbed cannabis cool to room temperature and then wrap in cheesecloth.

6. Fill a mason jar with either 16 ounces of oil or melted butter (and some water). The level of the oil or butter should be such that it is covered by the water in the sous vide. Submerge the cheesecloth in the oil or butter and secure the lid.

7. Check that the sous vide water is heated to 200°F.

8. Place the jar into the sous vide, taking care that the oil or butter is under water, but the lid is not. Heat the jar for 60 to 90 minutes.

9. Every 15 minutes, open the jar and press the cheesecloth to the side of the jar using a spoon, releasing the cannabis and ensuring every bit is used.

10. After about an hour, remove the jar and let it cool. Take the cheesecloth bag out and squeeze it one last time.

11. Strain oil/butter through a strainer lined with cheesecloth into a clean jar.

12. Mark your infusion with potency (see below) and strain (Wolf 2013).

Calculating Potency: Resources and Basic Math

Figuring out the potency of your infused products can be slightly difficult, but you want to make sure that you are doing it correctly, because this is how you determine dosages. We will start from the beginning, and then we'll point out some shortcuts.

Since olive oil is a healthy, versatile ingredient used in many cannabis-infused recipes, we'll use an infusion of 2 cups of olive oil as our example.

Start with 7 grams (¼ ounce) of cannabis flower. Choose a strain that has a potency of 15% THC (or CBD). Use 2 cups of high-quality extra-virgin olive oil.

When you follow the infusion instructions provided, your 2 cups of infused olive oil will have a potency of 25 milligrams of THC (or CBD) per tablespoon and 8 milligrams of THC (or CBD) per teaspoon. If your recipe called for 2 tablespoons of infused oil and provided four servings, each serving would have a 12.5% dose of THC (or CBD). Yes, it takes a bit of practice to get your numbers right, but once you do, you can determine what dose works for you. Of course, if you don't want to do these calculations yourself, you can visit OurCommunityHarvest.com/calculator. Plug in potency, amount of cannabis flower, amount of oil, how many teaspoons the recipe calls for, and numbers of servings. Easy as infused pie!

Homegrown Bud

If you home grow, even if you knew the potency of the plant, seed, or clone that resulted in your bud, the final potency of your harvest may be quite different. There are so many variables that the end product's potency will be nearly impossible to predict. In this case, use caution and calculate your infusion at 10% THC and/or CBD. Then, you'll have to try the infusion—at a very low dose—and figure out how close your calculations were. And I definitely would not serve the infused oil to any one else until I figured out its approximate potency.

tCheck2

If you really want to push the easy button, purchase one of these devices. The newest version of the device, the tCheck2, will test raw bud, infused butters and oils, and alcohol tinctures.

The tCheck2.
Know the potency
of your cannabis,
tinctures, and oils
with the tCheck2.

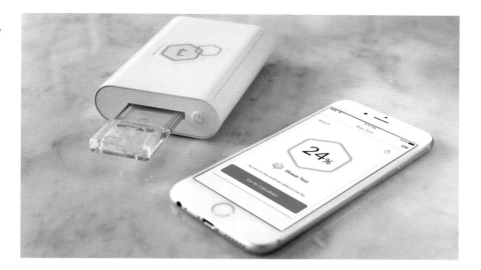

Devices for Decarboxylating and Infusing

If the thought of decarboxylating, slow simmering, and dosing your infused oil or butter strikes you as a hassle, there are a couple of very good, specialized devices you can use. We'll cover the Nova, the Levo, and the MagicalButter MB2e.

Here is the rationale home cannacook Corinne Tobias uses when considering the use of specialized cannabis devices: "I . . . only recommend gadgets . . . that:

1. I use every time I make cannabis infusions.
2. Make my edibles more potent or easier to make/dose.
3. I would recommend to a cranky relative on a fixed income (i.e.,

they're objectively worth the cost because of the service they provide or the money they save).
4. I would replace using my own cash money if I broke it.
5. In short, if it makes my life easier or edibles better . . . I'm excited to share it with you."

Here is what Corinne had to say about the Nova, the Levo, and the MagicalButter MB2e (I have added some transitional information as well).

Decarboxylating: The Nova

The Nova is the first thing Corinne recommends to folks who are looking to make infused medicine at home. In lab testing, the Nova transformed 100% of THCA to THC. These tests also showed that Corinne was losing

A GATEWAY TO GOOD HEALTH

CORINNE TOBIAS, *Functional Cannabis Coach and Cannabis Cookbook Author*

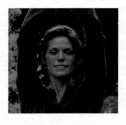

When I was 18, I was diagnosed with degenerative disc disease, scoliosis, herniated discs, and ADHD. Throughout my teens and 20s, I tried every diet, pain relief technique, and pill on the market; I was still in pain, depressed, unmotivated, fat, and cynical.

I had tried cannabis before, but because I was overweight, I hated the munchies and didn't like doing it often. In 2007, I was just curious and poor enough that I stumbled onto microdosing. I used a one-hitter to make my cannabis last longer and would get just the right effect to want to walk around for hours, drink a lot of water, and do a bunch of yoga.

For me, cannabis was a gateway drug. It was the gateway to a healthier and more vibrant lifestyle. It took several years to really get to a good place with my health because I didn't really know what I was doing, and I stumbled a lot along the way. When I figured out how this health thing worked, I decided to become a wellness blogger and yoga teacher, and later a health coach, incorporating cannabis so I could share how this beautiful plant could really help people.

As a functional cannabis coach, my mission is to change the way people see cannabis

after all of these years of prohibition. I want everyone to understand exactly how cannabis can help restore balance in your body and accelerate changes in your life that you've been dying to make.

I'm sure that to some, I'm one of those annoying "I did it and so can you!!" people, but in my defense: I did. And you can.

After writing about cannabis for years, I finally feel like I've found my purpose by incorporating cannabis with my other health and wellness work. I love working with clients to help them transform their health and their lives without running into all of the stumbling blocks I ran into along the way. I live to do this. Waking up and seeing other people do such incredible work for themselves and see how that actually is making the world a better place is the most rewarding thing I've ever done with my time.

I'm here to educate patients, doctors, and family members so they know that there are effective alternatives to many prescription drugs. I'm here to empower my clients, readers, and students so they know they can change their lives and take care of their bodies and create lives that they love waking up to. And I'm here to defeat this damned stigma and help end prohibition once and for all.

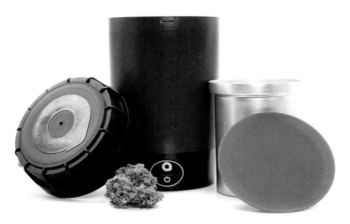

The Nova. The sleek Nova decarboxylates/slow roasts your cannabis with no odor and preserves the plant's potency, preparing it for infusing.

about 33% of her THC using the oven method—which means if she decarbed a pound of cannabis, she wasted ⅓ of a pound. BUM. MER.

If you're using edibles or tinctures as your primary medicine, and you want to save money by making more potent and active oil using less material, the Nova decarboxylator does that. Plus, the Nova is airtight, so it doesn't smell at all, and it also works with CBD-dominant strains. Corinne uses it every single time she cooks; after making her first batch, she was able to cut the dose in half.

Infusers

Corinne and I will now turn our attention to the Levo versus the MagicalButter MB2e. When it comes to making cannabis infusions, temperature is most of the battle. However, if you're making cannabis infusions as your primary medicine, you may also want to consider cleanup, ease of use, and quality of the end product.

Corinne has done years of "kitchen testing" and has never met a slow cooker, oven, or stovetop burner that can do what these two gadgets do. She temperature-tested every conventional device she owned, and even on warm or a set temperature, the temperature of the oil fluctuates.

Enter the Levo and the Magical Butter MB2e. These herbal infusers are great at holding a set temperature over extended periods of time, which makes them ideal for cannabis infusions.

They're very different machines, and if you're trying to decide which one to add to your bag of tricks, you'll have to consider your needs: frequency of use, volume of material you're infusing, how much scratch is in your wallet, and types of infusions you'd like to make.

LEVO

The LEVO is a great countertop device for making small-batch infusions. If you don't grow your own cannabis and buy it by the ounce (or less), or if you prefer to make small batches of infused oil, the LEVO is perfect. It uses an infusion method that doesn't pulverize your herb, and dispenses infused oil directly into a jar or container, making it the cleanest infusion method I've ever used. Since the LEVO gently infuses your oil or butter, it doesn't whip in any air bubbles, which increases the shelf life of your oil. I compared the potency of this oil with the other oils I've made throughout this book and it was just as potent as any other method, but had the best flavor.

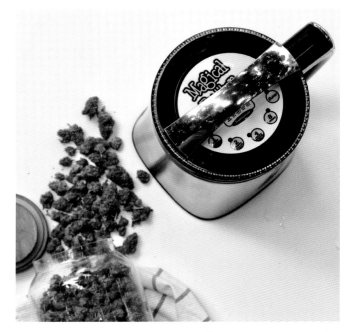

MagicalButter MB2e. When you are infusing a large amount of cannabis or want to make salves, sauces, and drinks, the MB2e is your go-to.

The gist: If you want to create the highest quality artisanal oils that will last for a long time, with the least amount of mess and the most control over temperature, the Levo was made for you. Plus, it is flat-out sleek and beautiful.

MagicalButter MB2e

On the other hand, the MagicalButter MB2e is great for processing a lot of material at one time and has been a staple in Corinne's kitchen for years. If you grow your own medicine and have

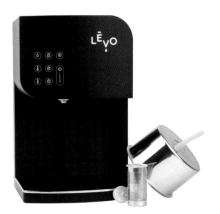

The LEVO. The Levo is ideal for small batch infusing and clean up is a cinch.

Infusing Section Summary

* Infusing oils and butters: Choose preferred strain and quantity.

* Inspect your cannabis for mold and discard if mold is detected.

* Crumble and decarb on low heat at about 200°F for about 60 minutes.

* Simmer in butter/oil for about 90 minutes.

* Strain, cool, and properly store your oil/butter.

* Terpenes and flavonoids contribute to the flavor and smell of cannabis.

* The entourage effect posits that the effect of the whole plant is better than its component parts.

* With edibles, go low and slow.

* Use the OurCommunityHarvest.com dosing calculator.

* Store infused butter/oil in cool, dark place.

DID YOU KNOW?

To promote her "Just Say No" campaign, Nancy Reagan appeared on the NBC sitcom *Different Strokes*? When compared to marijuana-based television shows of today, that episode, along with other stereotypical marijuana classics like *Three's Company*, show how far television has come in portraying the legality and legitimacy of marijuana.

a lot of material to turn into infusions at the end of the season or cycle, the MB2e is perfect. Keep in mind that, unlike the LEVO, you can't make small batches.

You'll need at least ½ ounce of cannabis and 2 cups of oil or butter to reach the minimum fill line. You can process up to 3 ounces of cannabis in 5 cups of oil, so it handles large amounts of post-harvest trim like a champion. It's also messier than the LEVO since you still have to strain the oil by hand, but it comes with a 90-micron filter and a silicone glove that make processing and straining very easy. As an added bonus, you can also make salves, tinctures, sauces, and drinks right in the device. It helps contain the smell when you're infusing oils, salves, and tinctures, and lights up your room like a disco party. The MB2e is Corinne's cannabis-processing workhorse.

The MagicalButter MB2e is a great high-volume infuser that can help you process your harvest quickly and easily. It's also awesome for whipping up tinctures and salves at a controlled temperature.

Chapter 6

INFUSED RECIPES FOR DAILY HEALTH & RECREATION

Now that you know how to infuse food, you can become your best health advocate by preparing a variety of recipes throughout the day. Depending on your goals, you may want to start your day with an infusion; perhaps you need a mid-day pick-up; or might want to prepare a healthy dinner. We have a number of recipe choices for you.

If you find that you want to infuse on a regular basis and want more recipes, there are several excellent cannabis cookbooks out there. A couple of our favorites are *Herb* by Chef Laurie Wolf and Melissa Parks. Wolf has written four different cannabis cookbooks and has been writing recipes for magazines for years, so she knows what she is doing. And Jessica Catalano's *The Ganja Kitchen Revolution* has an interesting take on pairing strains that have strong flavor profiles, like lemon, lavender, and mushroom, with complementary foods. Jessica hosts infused dinners on a regular basis, so she too knows how to explain infusing and offers creative, fun recipes. And of course, Corinne Tobias' *Wake and Bake* and *Dazed and Infused* cookbooks are entertaining and full of healthful advice and tips.

Dosing

Dosing is very important. The first step is to know the potency of your ingredients (see page 98 on how to determine potency).

Take a look at the table at right to get an idea of how microdoses in an edible compare to wine or smoking cannabis.

Trial and Error

Probably the most popular (although not the most recommended) way to know your dose is to try something and just wait. As you recall, it takes 30 minutes to 2 hours for the edibles to take effect, and then the effects often last from 4 to 8 hours—which means the whole experience may take up to 10 hours. When Corinne was writing her first cookbook, that's all she did: She made edibles; she ate edibles; she waited for the edibles to kick in, and took detailed notes. It was the best gig she could dream up at the time and she really liked the "testing" part of making those books, until one fateful day, a cannabis-infused grilled cheese took her out. She was unable to function; while it was transformative and illuminating, it was not fun.

MICRODOSING GUIDE

Quantity	Approximate Wine Equivalent	Ballpark Smoking Equivalent
2.5 mg of a sativa infusion	½ to ⅔ glass of red wine	1 good puff or 2
5 mg of a sativa infusion	1 to 1 ¼ glasses of red wine	About 2 to 3 puffs
7.5 mg of a sativa infusion	About 2 glasses of red wine	4 to 5 puffs
10 mg of a sativa infusion	2 ½ to 3 glasses of red wine	¾ of a joint or more

Note: Remember that an indica infusion lends itself to relaxation and often sleep while a sativa infusion often spurs energy, creativity, laughter, and sociability. And while the effects of alcohol and smoking cannabis differ in key ways from eating edibles, I wanted to give new and newish users at least a starting point to think about the results of edibles.

Accurate Measuring

Shortly after that, someone told Corinne about the tCheck (page 98), and she's been using that to test her oils ever since. The tCheck2 can easily help you regulate your dose so you don't have to be a human guinea pig.

A Word About Microdosing

If you can usually handle 10% THC in edibles at once, but have a four-course meal with 2.5% THC in each, over the course of the evening you may feel the effects more strongly; in some diners, the small doses seem to build on each other to become greater than the total. But conversely, microdosing is better for some, because you can feel and appreciate the effects on a gradual basis. So, go low (with the dosage) and slow if you try edibles. It may take you up to 2 hours to feel any effects, so be patient. And even if you metabolize quickly, you won't feel edibles for around 30 minutes. There also seems to be no correlation between height/weight and level of fitness with regards to feeling the effects of edibles. So, assuming a larger person can consume more edibles may not be true. As with all of the cannabis options available, you'll have to figure out what works for you.

Cooking with a CBD Infusion

Apparently, THC can handle a bit more heat than CBD, which means that lower temperatures are kinder to CBD infusions. When you use your CBD oil, it is recommended you don't heat it to temperatures above 240°F. So, we find CBD to be especially useful for sauces, to drizzle on foods that are served at room temperature, to add to beverages, and for salad dressings. Or serve it after the food is cooked and still warm. For example, you wouldn't want to put CBD oil in a pizza recipe that needs to go into a 450°F oven, but once the pizza cooled, you could certainly drizzle some oil on a piece or two.

Terpenes and Flavonoids

Many cannabis chefs like to pair the flavor and smell of particular cannabis strains that they believe complement the dish they are preparing. For example, if you were making a drizzle for seafood, you may want to use a cannabis strain that smells and tastes a bit like lemons. But, if you are careful when you make your infusions, you can almost eliminate the taste of cannabis so your butter and oil taste simply like, well, butter and oil.

Terpenes and flavonoids are, in the simplest sense, the flavors, tastes, colors, and smells of cannabis. When you cook with cannabis, you may taste and smell some of the strongest components of the strain; they'll add to your enjoyment when you match the right strain and dish. Some of the smells, tastes, and colors from terpenes and flavonoids include lemon, pine, mushroom, lavender, and mint; colors include deep green, yellow, light brown, purple, and even pink!

Last Notes on Cooking

You may remember a concept called The Entourage Effect, which was suggested by Raphael Mechoulam. The theory is that some cannabis compounds have seemingly no effect on their own, but when combined with other cannabis chemical compounds, can affect the human body in unique ways. Since there are more than 400 chemical compounds in cannabis, it may take a while for science to figure out how all the compounds work together, but for now it is thought the whole plant is more beneficial than particular parts of the plant. This means that when you cook with or consume cannabis, you should use as much of the full plant as you can.

This is also an appropriate time to remind the reader about combining alcohol with edible cannabis. This is also a case of the total being greater than the sum of its parts. In other words, if you can usually drink two large glasses of wine with dinner and feel fine, you may not feel the same way if you have an infused cannabis meal. The alcohol interacts with the cannabis and accelerates the potency of the THC. Edibles consumers who are also drinkers should either not combine alcohol with edibles or at least cut down their drinking by half.

Remember, you must pay attention to dosing, which will require you to do a lot of sometimes tricky math. You may have to convert teaspoons, ounces, grams, milligrams, metric units, imperial units, and more. So, make sure to have a calculator and possibly a scale nearby, or make it as easy as possible and use the calculator at OurCommunityHarvest.com/calculator.

Have separate cookware for your cannabis. A sharp knife, cutting board, measuring cups and spoons, a deep sauté pan, cheesecloth, labels, baking sheet for decarboxylation, a scale, wooden spoon, silicone ice cube tray, a strainer and mason jars for storage are all great items to dedicate to your cannabis creations.

Make sure to mark all infused butters, oils, and dishes clearly with date and potency.

Keep all of your infused products and your raw cannabis away from kids, animals, and adults who don't want to partake. You may even want to consider purchasing a stash box to keep your product safe and secure.

FLAVONOIDS

Flavonoids give vivid color to fruits, vegetables, flowers, and cannabis strains. In cannabis, they attract pollinators, work as a UV light filter, and repel pests. To date, we know about 20 flavonoids in cannabis. Here are some of the most beneficial.

Flavonoid	Benefits	Also Found In
Apigenin	Anti-inflammatory and antioxidant	Parsley and celery
Beta-sitosterol	Anti-inflammatory	Nuts and avocadoes
Kaempferol	Anti-depressant	Apples, grapes, and tomatoes
Orientin	Anti-aging, antioxidant, anti-inflammatory, anti-bacterial, painkiller; supports heart and brain health	Buckwheat and bamboo leaves
Quercetin	Antioxidant, fights viruses	Red wine, onions, and berries
Silymarin	Enhances liver function, protects liver	Milk thistle and wild artichokes
Vitexin and isovitexin	Encourages death of cancer cells (Ganesan and Xu 2017)	Passionflower and mung bean

PUFFIN MUFFIN FLAPJACKS

Ah—the smell of fresh pancakes in the morning is always a hit. These homemade Puffin Muffin Flapjacks are fluffy, filling, and delicious. For an extra kick, infused syrup will elevate your experience.

INGREDIENTS

2 tablespoons raw sugar

2½ tablespoons plus ½ cup flour

2 tablespoons infused coconut oil

1 egg

1 tablespoon agave, honey, or maple

½ cup nut milk

½ teaspoon baking soda

1 teaspoon baking powder

½ teaspoon vanilla extract

¼ cup blueberries (fresh, frozen, or dried)

Butter and syrup for serving

DIRECTIONS

In a small bowl, combine raw sugar and 2½ T flour; cut in infused coconut oil.

In a large bowl, whisk egg, agave, honey, or maple, nut milk, baking soda, baking powder, and vanilla extract.

Mix in ½ cup flour and the raw sugar mixture. Fold in blueberries.

Grease pan or griddle over medium-high heat.

Pour ¼ to ⅓ cup batter onto pan or griddle.

When bubbles appear in the middle and stay there, use a spatula to flip! Cook for 1 to 2 minutes on other side. Serve with butter and syrup.

Serves 6.

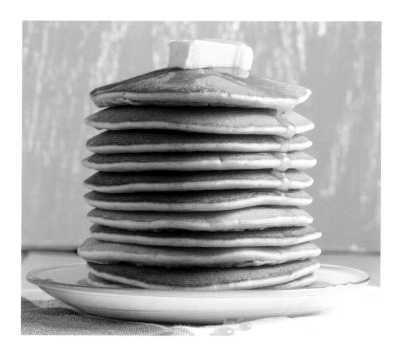

BULLSEYE EGG BAKE

I'm a big fan of eggs and this recipe hits the target every time. The star of this potato mashup is an eye-catching golden egg in the center. Vegetarians can substitute roasted vegetables for the egg as a healthy, delicious alternative. Yum!

INGREDIENTS

½ to ¾ cup mashed potato or sweet potato

1 teaspoon infused olive oil

1 egg or roasted vegetables

Salt and pepper

DIRECTIONS

Grease one large ramekin lightly. Preheat oven to 375°F.

In a cup or small bowl, combine mashed potato or sweet potato and infused olive oil.

Fill ¾ of the ramekin with mashed potato mixture.

Bake about 10 to 15 minutes, until potatoes are golden.

Remove ramekin from the oven and crack an egg (or layer roasted veggies) on the top of the potato mix. Sprinkle with salt and pepper.

Place ramekin back in the oven and bake until desired yolk solidness.

Serves 1.

FAKE BAKE CARROT CAKE MUFFINS

These tasty muffins will satisfy your sweet tooth while delivering the nutrition of a cup of carrots. To make them even more irresistible, consider adding walnuts.

INGREDIENTS

1 cup sugar

⅜ cup coconut oil (melted)

2 tablespoons infused coconut oil (melted)

2 eggs

1 cup flour

¼ teaspoon salt

½ teaspoon baking soda

½ teaspoon baking powder

½ teaspoon cinnamon

1 cup grated carrots

DIRECTIONS

Grease the wells of a muffin tin. Preheat oven to 350°F.

In a large bowl, mix sugar, melted coconut oil, melted infused coconut oil, and eggs.

In a medium bowl, whisk flour, salt, baking soda, baking powder, and cinnamon.

Slowly incorporate dry ingredients into wet ingredients.

Fold in grated carrots.

Scoop batter into muffin tin (wells should be ⅔ to ¾ full).

Bake until edges are golden and toothpick comes out cleanly.

Serves 4.

CLASSIC HAM AND CHEESE PANINI

It could be the crusty, gently fried bread, or the winning combination of ham and cheese that makes this recipe a favorite. Easy and quick to make, paninis pair well with soups and salads to round out a healthy, satisfying meal.

INGREDIENTS

1 small, hoagie-size roll or small loaf of French bread

1 teaspoon infused butter or oil

2 pieces of ham or prosciutto

2 pieces of cheese, such as swiss or provolone

Yellow mustard

Sliced pickles (optional)

DIRECTIONS

Cut bread in two and spread infused butter or oil on insides.

Layer two pieces of ham (or prosciutto, which makes a nice substitute), two pieces of cheese, mustard, and, if you prefer, pickles on the bread. Then place it in a panini press until golden brown. If you don't have a panini press, simply place the sandwich in a cast iron or heavy pan and place another heavy pan on top of it.

Check periodically, flip once, and remove from pan when golden brown and cheese is melted and gooey.

Serves 1.

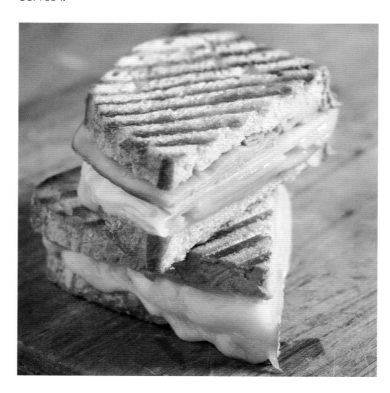

ROASTED VEGGIE QUICHE

Seasonal, roasted vegetables complemented by fresh herbs and delivered in a pie crust gives this Roasted Veggie Quiche its broad appeal. Equally tasty right out of the oven or eaten at room temperature, it's a great dish to make ahead and savor.

INGREDIENTS

1 large bell pepper

½ large onion

1 medium russet potato

2 tablespoons infused olive oil

1 to 2 tablespoons herbs (rosemary, thyme, or sage)

1 cup flour

½ teaspoon salt

6 tablespoons coconut oil, cold

2 tablespoons infused coconut oil, cold

3 to 4 tablespoons ice-cold water

6 to 7 eggs

DIRECTIONS

Preheat oven to 300°F.

Chop bell pepper, onion, and potato into ½-inch chunks.

In a medium bowl, toss chopped veggies with infused olive oil and herbs.

Spread veggie mixture onto a baking sheet and roast in the oven for 20 to 30 minutes, stirring occasionally.

While veggies are roasting, whisk flour and salt. Cut in coconut oil and cold infused coconut oil; mix in ice water to create the pie dough.

Lightly knead dough until it holds together.

Roll out pie dough on floured surface and fold in half. Put dough in pie tin, pierce the crust several times, or weigh down with pie weights and prebake in oven for about 10 minutes.

Scramble eggs and fold in roasted vegetables.

Pour egg and vegetable mixture into prebaked pie crust.

Bake until golden on top and when fork or knife inserted near center comes out clean.

Serves 6.

VEGETABLE SPRING ROLLS
with Dipping Sauce

Spring rolls are deceptively easy to make but stand out as beautiful, fresh appetizers. If this is your first time making the dipping sauce, go easy on the fish sauce, which has a strong, distinct taste.

INGREDIENTS

Spring Rolls:

1 package spring roll wrappers

1½ cups of your choice of mushrooms, carrots, red onions, bell peppers, or cabbage, chopped

8 to 12 pieces grilled (preferred) or boiled shrimp (optional)

Dipping Sauce:

⅓ cup low-sodium soy sauce

1 tablespoon infused olive oil

Juice of ½ lime or lemon

Dash of fish sauce

Pinch of sugar

1 teaspoon red pepper flakes

DIRECTIONS

Spring Rolls

Spring roll wrappers are rice wrappers that look like very thin, translucent tortillas, and can be found in grocery stores and specialty Asian groceries.

Prepare your choice of vegetables. You can use them raw or quickly sauté at this point. When making your selections, try to mix a crunchy vegetable with a soft one.

If using shrimp, clean and devein, brush with olive oil, and place directly on medium-hot grill. Grill 3 minutes per side and shrimp will turn pink and curl when done. If boiling, clean and devein, boil 2 quarts of water, boil shrimp for 3 minutes, and then place in cold water/ice water to stop the cooking process.

Put spring roll wrapper in warm water for 10 seconds or until pliable. Place softened spring roll wrapper on dry cutting board.

Put a spoonful of vegetable filling in middle of wrapper. Add shrimp, if using. Fold sides until they touch the filling. Roll from the back until it looks like a little burrito. Makes about 10 rolls that can be cut in half.

Serves about 6 to 8.

Dipping Sauce

Combine ingredients in small bowl. Dip spring roll in sauce as desired.

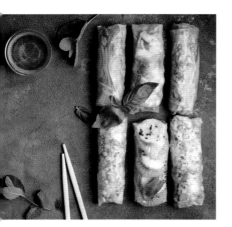

BOSTON LETTUCE SALAD
with *Almonds and Fresh Herbs*

A simple way to add more vegetables to your diet is to try this healthy, tasty salad that packs a zesty, herb kick. If you make extra dressing, be sure to label the dressing with potency and date and store with care.

INGREDIENTS

Salad:

⅓ cup sliced and roasted almonds

6 cups (1 large head) Boston or Bibb lettuce, torn

1 cup fresh parsley, chopped

½ cup fresh cilantro, chopped

¼ cup fresh chives, cut into ½-inch lengths

Vinaigrette:

2 tablespoons infused olive oil

2 tablespoons non-infused olive oil

1 tablespoon shallots

Juice of ½ lemon

DIRECTIONS

Preheat oven to 400°F.

Spread sliced almonds on cookie sheet and roast. Stir occasionally until golden, about 5 minutes. Remove almonds from oven and let cool to room temperature.

In a large bowl, toss torn lettuce, parsley, cilantro, and chives. Add roasted almond slices.

Whisk ingredients for vinaigrette and dress the salad.

Serves 4.

MIXED GREEN SALAD
with *Artichoke Heart Vinaigrette*

If you are pinched for time, this easy-to-make salad is perfect.
It contains few ingredients and goes well with any number of dishes.
The vinaigrette is surprisingly fresh and can be made in minutes.

INGREDIENTS

Salad:
4 cups mixed salad greens
   (romaine, iceberg, mesclun,
   or combine several salad
   greens)

Vinaigrette:
3 tablespoons fresh lemon
   juice

2 tablespoons infused
   olive oil

2 tablespoons non-infused
   olive oil

Pinch of salt and pepper

12 to 15-ounce jar marinated
   artichoke hearts

DIRECTIONS

In large bowl, toss mixed salad greens.

In small bowl, make the vinaigrette by whisking together all ingredients (except artichoke hearts).

Drain the marinated artichoke hearts, rinse them, and chop roughly. Add to vinaigrette.

Toss mixed greens with vinaigrette.

Serves 4.

TOMATO, OLIVE, CUCUMBER, AND FETA SALAD

With a toasted piece of pita bread on the side, this salad will make you feel like you are visiting the Greek islands. The sour-tasting feta, salty olives, juicy tomatoes, and cucumbers meld together in perfect harmony.

INGREDIENTS

Salad:

1 pound cherry tomatoes, halved

¾ pound cucumbers, rough-chopped

½ cup Kalamata olives, diced

½ cup crumbled feta cheese

¼ cup chopped fresh dill

Dressing:

2 tablespoons infused olive oil

6 tablespoons non-infused olive oil

4 tablespoons red wine vinegar

Pinch of sugar

1 garlic clove, minced

1 teaspoon dried oregano (or 1 tablespoon minced fresh)

Pinch of garlic powder

Pinch of salt and pepper

DIRECTIONS

Combine salad ingredients in large bowl and toss.

Whisk the dressing ingredients together and mix with salad. Place salad in refrigerator for 30 minutes to 2 hours.

Serves 4.

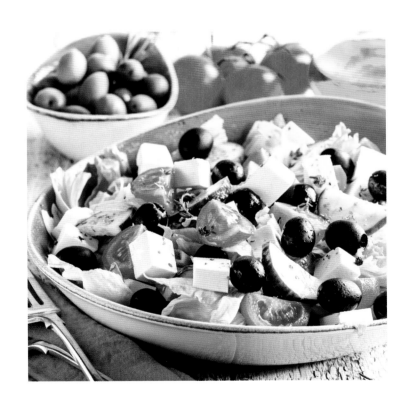

CORNBREAD WITH TOPPINGS

This cornbread is absolutely delicious by itself, but you won't go wrong eating it with a good chili. If you prefer crispy cornbread, as I do, make sure your batter only fills one inch (or less) of your cast iron skillet.

INGREDIENTS

Cornbread:

1½ cups cornmeal

2 cups milk, warmed

2 cups flour

1 tablespoon baking powder

1 teaspoon salt

¼ cup sugar

2 eggs

2 tablespoons infused butter, melted

⅜ cup non-infused vegetable oil

Vegetable oil or bacon fat (for greasing skillet)

Warm beans (for serving)

Pico de Gallo:

6 roma tomatoes

2 small jalapenos

1 medium red or white onion

2 cloves garlic, minced

½ bunch cilantro, chopped

1½ cups organic sweet corn (optional)

DIRECTIONS

Preheat oven to 400°F; while oven is preheating, place cast-iron skillet on stove top on low heat.

Combine cornmeal with warmed milk. Let soak for about 15 minutes.

In large bowl, mix flour, baking powder, salt, and sugar.

In moist cornmeal, whisk in eggs, melted infused butter, non-infused vegetable oil, and dry mixture; do not over-stir, as you want a few lumps to remain.

Barely cover the bottom of the cast-iron pan with vegetable oil (if you have bacon fat on hand, it is highly recommended to use it here!).

Pour the batter into the hot skillet (be careful, that cast-iron pan gets hot) and then place in oven using multiple hot pads.

Bake for 30 to 40 minutes until golden brown and a knife or fork inserted in the center comes out clean.

Pico de Gallo

Cut roma tomatoes and jalapenos in half. Squeeze the juice out of the tomatoes and remove the seeds from the jalapenos (the heat is in the seeds, so leave some if you'd like more heat).

Dice the roma tomatoes, the jalapenos, and the onion.

In a large bowl, mix all ingredients. Optional: Add organic sweet corn.

Refrigerate until chilled (flavor develops even more after a day or so).

When your cornbread has cooled down, cut into equal slices. Cover with warm beans and chilled pico de gallo.

Serves 6.

KALAMATA HUMINAHUMINA HUMMUS

*There is no question about it; hummus is in vogue as an appetizer.
This recipe combines a traditional ingredient, chickpeas,
with kalamata olives and capers for a unique mouthwatering taste.*

INGREDIENTS

⅓ cup tahini

Juice from 1 lemon

¾ cup kalamata olives, pitted

2 tablespoons capers (optional, but recommended)

2 tablespoons infused olive oil

16-ounce can garbanzo beans (chick peas), rinsed

Pinch of salt

Toasted pita bread or carrots, celery, and cucumbers for serving

Variation:
¾ cup roasted red pepper, chopped

2 tablespoons cumin

2 tablespoons garlic

DIRECTIONS

In a food processor, blend tahini and lemon juice until smooth.

Add the pitted kalamata olives, capers (if using), and infused olive oil.

Slowly add garbanzo beans ¼ cup at a time until you reach the desired consistency and flavor.

Season with salt to taste. Serve with toasted pita bread or carrots, celery, and cucumbers.

Serves 6.

For a variation, omit the olives and add chopped roasted red pepper, cumin, and garlic instead.

COCKTAIL MEATBALLS

Sweet, savory, and slightly spicy are the best ways to describe these party-favorite meatballs. They are one of the first dishes to disappear at a gathering. I adapted this from my mother-in-law's recipe.

INGREDIENTS

Meatballs:
1 pound ground beef

¾ cup rolled oats

½ cup milk

1 tablespoon Worcestershire sauce

½ teaspoon onion powder

Pinch of salt

Dash of hot sauce, such as Tabasco

2 tablespoons infused butter

Sauce:
¾ cup water

¾ cup vinegar

¾ cup sugar or pineapple juice

1 teaspoon paprika

2 teaspoons corn starch

1 tablespoon cold water

DIRECTIONS

In a large bowl, combine ingredients for meatballs.

Make individual meatballs about the size of a golf ball.

Brown the meatballs in a skillet over medium heat until cooked through, giving them some exterior color and texture.

Sauce for Cocktail Meatballs
In large sauce pan, add water, vinegar, sugar or pineapple juice, and paprika.

Simmer for 5 to 10 minutes. Combine corn starch with cold water and add to sauce. Let thicken and then place browned meatballs in sauce. Can be served warm or at room temperature.

Serves 6.

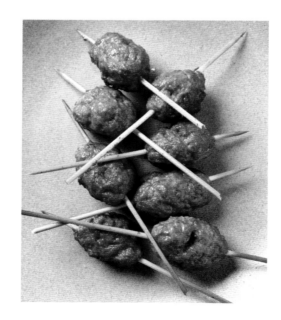

— Quick Ideas —

MOZZARELLA, TOMATO, AND BASIL BITE

Start with a slice of mozzarella. Top it with fresh, seasonal tomato slice and a fresh basil leaf. Drizzle with infused olive oil. Sprinkle with kosher salt and cracked black pepper. On the side, place a small piece of toasted French bread to sop up any extra oil.

BRUSCHETTA

Toast pieces of French bread and drizzle with infused olive oil. Top with chopped tomatoes, capers, red onion, and fresh parsley.

SCALLOPS

Season scallops with chili powder or Old Bay seasoning and place in medium-hot pan with butter or oil (non-infused). Cook about a minute and a half on both sides until brown. Place on a small bed of arugula or baby spinach and drizzle with infused olive oil.

SHRIMP

Peel and devein shrimp. Season with garlic, curry, cumin, and pepper and grill or sauté shrimp until pink and done. Place on a bed of seasonal greens and drizzle with infused olive oil.

GARLIC AND GOAT CHEESE TOAST

Chop off the top of a whole head of garlic and drizzle with non-infused olive oil. Place in preheated 350°F oven for 40 minutes, until soft. Cut loaf of French bread and slather each piece with this "garlic jam." Top with goat cheese and place back in oven for 5 minutes or until goat cheese is melted. Top with chopped walnuts and infused olive oil.

Side Dishes

BABY SPINACH SALAD

with *Strawberries and Walnuts*

This recipe combines strawberries and spinach with walnuts for crunch, cheese for a tangy lift, and quality balsamic vinegar to bring it all together. or an even bigger taste, boil and chop an egg and add to the salad party.

INGREDIENTS

Salad:

1 pound baby spinach

2 cups strawberries, chopped

½ cup crumbled glazed walnuts

2 to 4 ounces crumbled goat, feta, or gorgonzola cheese

1 red onion, thinly sliced

Vinaigrette:

3 tablespoons infused olive oil

1 tablespoon non-infused olive oil

1/2 cup balsamic vinegar

1 tablespoon honey

DIRECTIONS

Toss together salad ingredients.

Whisk together vinaigrette ingredients, then combine with salad and toss.

Serves 8.

THREE BEAN SALAD

A versatile vegetarian side dish, this protein-packed salad is a perfect dish to make ahead as a non-infused option. Then, if you or your guests want an infusion, you can add a bit of infused oil as needed.

INGREDIENTS

12-ounce can cannellini beans

12-ounce can chickpeas or black beans

12-ounce can kidney beans

1 tablespoon lemon juice

1½ teaspoons rosemary, minced

2 tablespoons non-infused olive oil

Pinch of salt and pepper

DIRECTIONS

Combine ingredients. This side works well with many meat dishes. When preparing, go easy on the olive oil and then add additional olive oil for those who don't want an infusion and some infused olive oil for those who do want another microdose.

Serves 8 to 10.

GAZPACHO

Start with good, local tomatoes, add crunchy vegetables, and serve with a piece of toasted French bread. I always make extra; this dish can be made a day or two ahead of time and is best served chilled.

INGREDIENTS

½ cup red wine vinegar

½ cup non-infused olive oil

2 cups canned tomato juice or V-8

3 eggs

2 red, yellow, or orange bell peppers

2 onions

2 large shallots

2 large cucumbers

6 ripe tomatoes

Dash of cayenne pepper or hot smoked paprika

Dash of salt and pepper

½ cup chopped fresh dill

Infused olive oil

French bread for serving

DIRECTIONS

Whisk together red wine vinegar, olive oil, tomato juice or V-8, and eggs. Use a food processor or blender to puree the vegetables in small batches, being sure to retain some of the crunch. Stir in a pinch of cayenne pepper (or hot smoked paprika) and salt and pepper to taste. Finally, add chopped fresh dill and then chill for at least two hours (overnight is even better). Add a drizzle of carefully dosed infused olive oil to an individual serving of the gazpacho and serve with a crunchy piece of French bread.

Serves 8 to 10.

— *Quick Ideas* —

MIXED GREEN SALAD

Dress with a traditional olive oil and vinegar dressing, substituting infused olive oil.

ROASTED SEASONAL VEGETABLES

Toss cubed root vegetables, such as carrots, potatoes, turnips, squash, parsnips, or sweet potatoes with olive oil, salt, pepper, and a couple pinches of rosemary. Roast in a 375°F oven for about 30 minutes or until vegetables are a little soft. Before serving, drizzle with infused olive oil.

BUTTERNUT SQUASH MASHUP

This recipe appears courtesy of my brother, Shatta, who enjoys his vegetables. He infuses individual portions by adding a precise amount of infused butter or olive oil prior to serving; be sure to mix well.

INGREDIENTS

1 medium butternut squash

1 clove garlic

2 parsnips

2 to 3 heirloom carrots

1 large turnip

2 small gold beets

1 cup chopped cauliflower

3 tablespoons infused olive oil

1 tablespoon non-infused olive oil, plus more for sautéing

Pinch of Himalayan coarse salt

Pinch of white pepper

Pinch of smoked paprika

Pinch of cayenne pepper

2 stalks rosemary

1/3 to 1/2 cup white wine

1/4 cup chopped white onion

1 to 2 sage leaves, minced

Juice of 1 lemon

3/4 cup heavy cream

1/2 cup crumbled gorgonzola cheese

1/4 cup smoked, roasted, salted, chopped almonds

3 sprigs parsley

DIRECTIONS

Heat oven to 450°F.

Halve the butternut squash. Remove ends, seeds, and skin, and cut into 1-inch pieces. Cut garlic cloves in half. Peel parsnips, carrots, turnip, and beets and cut into 1-inch pieces. Cut cauliflower into 1-inch pieces as well. Put all cut vegetables into large bowl, add olive oil, salt, pepper, paprika, cayenne pepper, and rosemary stalks, and stir to coat well.

Add about 1/3 cup white wine (enough to cover the bottom) to a baking dish and add vegetables. Roast in oven for 30 to 40 minutes until vegetables are cooked through. Stir the vegetables once while they are roasting and add more white wine if liquid has evaporated. While vegetables are roasting, sauté onions and sage on stovetop for about 5 minutes or until onions are translucent.

When vegetables are roasted, place in mixing bowl with sautéed onions, sage, lemon juice, and heavy cream. Mash by hand or blend until you reach desired consistency. Top with gorgonzola, almonds, and parsley to serve.

Serves 6 to 8.

SIMPLE CRAB CAKES
with *Easy Ancho Sauce*

In my opinion, a good crab cake is made with a minimum of mayonnaise and bread crumbs; use just enough to bind the patties. It also helps to chill the raw cakes for a few minutes before baking. Serve on a bed of baby spinach or mixed greens.

INGREDIENTS

Crab Cakes:

1 pound crab meat, divided in half

1 lightly beaten egg

Scant 1/3 cup mayonnaise

1/2 cup panko bread crumbs

2 tablespoons infused olive oil

2 teaspoons Worcestershire sauce

2 tablespoons Dijon mustard

Pinch of smoked paprika or cayenne pepper

Pinch of salt and pepper

Greens or bread for serving

Ancho Sauce:

7-ounce (or smaller) can ancho peppers in sauce

1/4 cup mayonnaise

DIRECTIONS

Preheat oven to 375°F.

In large bowl, combine the first half of the crab meat with the other ingredients. Gently fold in the rest of the crab until it just holds together. Only add enough panko to bind the crab cake.

Shape into 4 to 6 cakes about an inch thick or less and place on lightly greased cookie sheet. Bake for 12 to 15 minutes. Flip crab cakes and bake for an additional 10 to 15 minutes until golden brown.

To make an easy ancho sauce, simply mince a quarter of an ancho pepper, mix with an additional teaspoon of ancho sauce, and combine with the mayonnaise. Most of the can of ancho peppers will not be used and can be saved for other recipes

Serve crab cakes on a bed of greens or make a sandwich using ancho sauce as a spread.

Serves 4 to 6.

Dinner/Winding Down Eats

NO-RISE, QUICK PIZZA

After you practice a few times, you can have a delicious homemade pizza on your table in about 30 minutes. Start a quick sauce, and while it is simmering, make your dough. To add more protein, as I do for my vegetarian son, add 3 tablespoons chia seeds. Just remember that the chia seeds will require more warm water.

INGREDIENTS

Pizza Sauce:

15-ounce can tomato sauce

1 teaspoon onion powder

1 teaspoon garlic powder

2 teaspoons oregano

Pinch of rosemary

2 teaspoons parsley

1 teaspoon sugar

⅛ cup red wine

Crust:

2¾ cups flour

1/4 cup cornmeal

3 tablespoons chia seeds
   (optional)

2 tablespoons infused
   olive oil

2 tablespoons baking powder

Pinch of salt

⅓ to ¾ cup warm water

Toppings:

2 cups mozzarella cheese

Other desired toppings,
   such as mushrooms, olives,
   sausage, pepperoni, ham

DIRECTIONS

Preheat oven to 450°F. To make the sauce, put ingredients in large pan and simmer for at least 15 to 25 minutes.

While sauce is simmering, make crust. In large bowl combine ingredients with enough water (adding a bit at a time) to bind. Dough should feel silky, but not sticky. If sticky, add a bit of flour, 1 tablespoon at a time. Let the dough rest for a few minutes at room temperature or place in refrigerator. Roll out and place in cast-iron pan or on cookie sheet.

Sprinkle some mozzarella cheese on bottom of crust. Top cheese with pizza sauce, additional toppings, and remainder of mozzarella cheese. Bake for 10 to 15 minutes until cheese is melted and crust is crispy.

Serves 4.

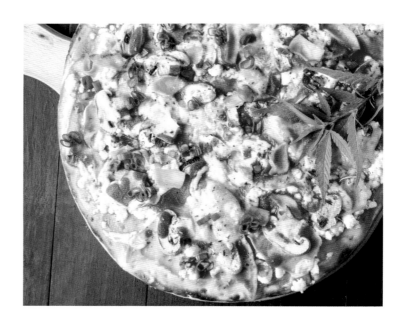

UDON NOODLES
with Veggies in Veggie Broth

Recently, both warm and cold noodle bowls have become quite popular. This simple version is a great place to start. When you master this recipe, feel free to add braised beef or pork, fried tofu cubes, or more and different vegetables.

INGREDIENTS

- 2 cups udon noodles
- ½ cup vegetables (your choice of yellow or green onion, celery, carrots, broccoli, mushrooms, peppers)
- 2 cloves garlic
- 2 tablespoons peanut oil (or vegetable oil)
- Pinch of ginger powder
- 1 tablespoon soy sauce
- 1 teaspoon sesame oil
- 2 tablespoons infused olive oil (or infused coconut oil)
- ½ cup vegetable stock
- Black sesame seeds for serving

DIRECTIONS

Udon noodles can be frozen or dry. Prepare following package directions.

Chop your choice of vegetables and 2 cloves of garlic. Sauté vegetables for about 5 minutes in peanut or vegetable oil with a pinch of powdered ginger, the soy sauce, and the sesame oil. Remove from pan, place in large bowl, drizzle infused olive or coconut oil on vegetables, and stir.

Heat vegetable stock until simmering. Take off heat, add noodles and vegetables to stock, and stir. Serve in individual bowls and garnish with black sesame seeds.

Serves 5.

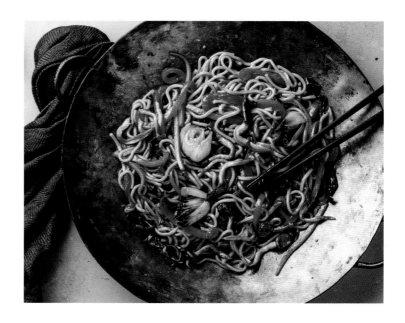

Dinner/Winding Down Eats

SOY MARINATED CHICKEN THIGHS
with *Lemon Zest*

My wife could eat chicken every day, and this recipe ranks as one of her favorites. Marinate the chicken for at least an hour, but preferably overnight. You will be rewarded with chicken that is crispy on the outside with a tasty, tangy flavor.

INGREDIENTS

4 tablespoons low-sodium soy sauce

2 tablespoons infused olive oil

2 garlic cloves, minced

1 tablespoon lemon or orange juice (save zest for plating)

1 teaspoon sesame oil

1 teaspoon brown sugar

8 chicken thighs

Black sesame seeds for serving

Green onion, thinly sliced for serving

DIRECTIONS

Combine ingredients (all but those for serving) in a large zip top bag. Marinate at least 1 hour and preferably up to 24 hours, shaking or turning every so often.

Preheat grill to medium heat. Remove thighs from bag and discard marinade. Place chicken on oiled grill for 5 to 10 minutes per side until internal temperature reaches at least 165°F.

When plating, add some zest to each thigh with some black sesame seeds and thin green onion pieces on top of the thighs which makes for a nice presentation.

Serves 4.

Note: If you do not have a grill, brown thighs on stovetop and finish in oven until internal temperature reaches at least 165°F. Be sure to oil your pan.

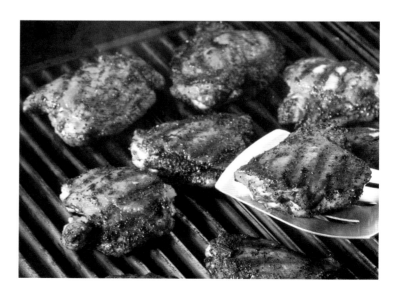

VEGETABLE LASAGNA

Feeding a crowd is a snap when you serve made-ahead vegetable lasagna.

INGREDIENTS

Vegetable oil spray

1 package no-boil
   lasagna noodles

Tomato Sauce:

1 28-ounce can crushed
   tomatoes

1 teaspoon onion powder

1 teaspoon garlic powder

⅓ cup fresh basil

Pinch of black pepper

Cream Sauce:

1 15-ounce container
   ricotta cheese

2 eggs

Pinch of nutmeg

¼ cup cream (optional)

Vegetable Filling:

1 cup sliced mushrooms

1 cup chopped bell peppers

1 onion, diced

2 heads of garlic, minced

2 tablespoons infused
   olive oil

1 cup chopped zucchini or
   eggplant (optional)

Topping/Cheese Filling:

2 cups shredded
   mozzarella cheese

½ cup shredded
   parmesan cheese

DIRECTIONS

Preheat oven to 375°F. Spray a 9 x 13-inch pan with vegetable oil.

For tomato sauce, simply stir ingredients together in a large bowl.

To make the cream sauce, beat eggs in a large bowl. Add the ricotta cheese to the eggs a little at a time until creamy. If it looks too grainy, add the cream. Put in pinch of nutmeg when you've reached your desired consistency.

To prepare the vegetable filling, sauté mushrooms, peppers, and onion in infused olive oil for about 5 minutes or until onions are translucent and vegetables have released much of their liquid. Sauté garlic separately for about 2 minutes and then add to the rest of vegetables. (If you skip this step and just use raw vegetables, you risk making a soggy lasagna). If you use eggplant or zucchini, chop into ½-inch cubes, wrap in paper towel, and press between two pans to remove moisture. Microwave for one minute and then sauté with the other vegetables.

Assemble your lasagna by spooning enough tomato sauce to cover bottom of the pan. Cover sauce with lasagna sheets. Spread a layer of cream sauce and layer of vegetable filling on lasagna sheets. Sprinkle some mozzarella and parmesan on top. Add another layer of lasagna sheets, cream sauce, vegetable filling, cheese, and top with lasagna sheets. Ladle tomato sauce on top and sprinkle rest of cheese. Place in oven and bake until cheese is melted and lasagna is golden brown and bubbling, about 25 to 35 minutes. Let cool and serve.

Serves 6.

Dinner/Winding Down Eats

SKIRT STEAK DRIZZLED
with *Chimichurri Sauce*

*When I visited my brother in Uruguay, we ate steak—lots of steak.
One of my favorite preparations was skirt steak drizzled with
garlicky, spicy, mouth-watering chimichurri sauce. This magical
sauce can also be used as a marinade and is easy to dose.*

INGREDIENTS

Steak:

1½ to 1¾ pounds skirt steak
(about ¾ to 1 inch thick)

Pinch of salt and pepper

Chimichurri Sauce:

1/2 cup non-infused
extra-virgin olive oil plus
2 tablespoons infused
olive oil

½ cup white or
red wine vinegar

3 garlic cloves, minced

1 small jalapeño,
finely chopped

½ cup minced fresh cilantro

⅓ cup minced fresh
flat-leaf parsley

2 tablespoons minced
fresh oregano

DIRECTIONS

Heat grill to medium high.

Pat skirt steak dry with paper towel and liberally season with salt
and pepper. Set aside and allow to come to room temperature.

In a small serving bowl, whisk together olive oil, vinegar, garlic,
jalapeño, cilantro, parsley, oregano, and a pinch of salt.

Grill steak about 3 minutes per side for medium rare. Let steak
rest for 10 minutes and then cut 1-inch pieces across the grain.
Put chimichurri sauce on table and drizzle as desired.

Serves 4 to 6.

FISH IN PARCHMENT PAPER
on a Bed of *White Beans, Arugula, Cherry Tomatoes, Garlic, and Sausage*

This upscale, restaurant-quality recipe makes use of parchment paper; the results are impressive and delicious. Each bite offers a unique combination of fish, vegetables, garlic, and spicy sausage with a little bit of broth. Serve with a toasted pieceof French bread so diners can sop up every bit of goodness.

INGREDIENTS

- 1 pound chorizo or hot sausage
- 2 tablespoons non-infused olive oil
- 3 cups arugula
- 15-ounce can northern white beans (preferred) or butter beans, rinsed
- 1 pint cherry tomatoes, halved
- 3 garlic cloves, halved
- 6 6-ounce pieces of white fish such as cod, haddock, or pollock
- 6 teaspoons infused olive oil
- Pinch of salt and pepper
- 1 loaf French bread for serving

DIRECTIONS

Preheat oven to 400°F.

Chop chorizo or hot sausage into ¼-inch cubes and cook until almost done. Set aside.

With non-infused olive oil, sauté arugula, white beans, halved cherry tomatoes, and halved garlic cloves. Stir often and when arugula begins to wilt, add chorizo or sausage and sauté another minute. Set aside and allow to cool.

Cut 6 sheets of parchment paper into 14-inch squares and place the first piece on a cookie sheet. Spoon about ½ cup of the arugula mixture in the center of the sheet. Place fish on arugula mixture, drizzle with 1 teaspoon infused olive oil, season with salt and pepper, and fold over parchment. Tightly crimp the edges until you've made a half moon shape and place on another cookie sheet; you should be able to fit 2 to 4 crimped pieces on each cookie sheet. Repeat until all 6 pieces of fish are enclosed in parchment paper.

Cook in oven for about 15 minutes. Toast a piece or two of French bread for each dish. Serve in a large soup bowl and garnish with the French bread. There, you've cooked with parchment!

Serves 6.

Drinks

THE GREEN DRINK

(a.k.a. The Green, Healthy Smoothie)

At first blush, a green drink may look strange, but after one serving your body will thank you. Low in calories, high in antioxidants, and packed with vitamins, this mean green smoothie will keep you hydrated and happy.

INGREDIENTS

2 large leaves of kale or chard

1 apple (green or slightly sour apples work best)

¼ cup parsley

¼ cup celery

1 teaspoon lemon juice (or apple cider vinegar)

1 teaspoon chia seeds (optional, but recommended)

2 cups water

1 teaspoon infused coconut oil, melted

DIRECTIONS

In a high-speed blender, combine all ingredients except infused coconut oil.

While blending, drizzle in the infused coconut oil.

Serve immediately.

Serves 1 to 2.

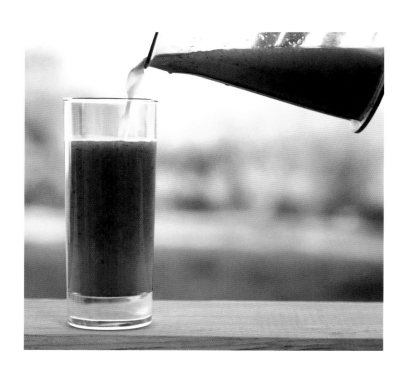

MATCHAJUANA DRINK
(Infused, Healthy Matcha Tea)

For centuries matcha tea has been used in Japanese tea ceremonies. Recently, it has been getting positive press for its healthy antioxidant and metabolism-boosting properties. This simple recipe gets a boost from infused coconut oil, which pairs surprisingly well.

INGREDIENTS

1 cup non-dairy milk (hemp, coconut, and almond milk work well)

1 cup hot water (or cold if you're making it iced)

2 teaspoons matcha tea

1 teaspoon infused coconut oil, melted

DIRECTIONS

In a blender, combine ingredients.

Blend and sweeten to taste.

Serves 2.

KEY LIME PIE INFUSED MILKSHAKE

Every time I make this, I can't help but sing "You put the lime in the coconut." And yes, you will drink it all up—happily! As a perfect summertime dessert, it will help you feel you are on vacation even if you are only sitting on your back porch.

INGREDIENTS

2 tablespoons key lime juice (Nellie & Joe's if possible)

2 tablespoons sugar

2 tablespoons milk

2 cups vanilla ice cream

1 teaspoon lime zest

2 tablespoons infused coconut oil

1 graham cracker for serving

Lime zest for serving (optional)

Lime wedge for serving

DIRECTIONS

In a blender, combine ingredients except graham cracker. Blend to desired consistency.

Crush a graham cracker and use crumbs as garnish. Use additional lime zest if you like.

Serve immediately with a reusable or recyclable straw and wedge of lime for decoration.

Serves 2 to 4.

Drinks

ADIRONDACK CHAIR HOMEMADE LEMONADE

Is there anything more symbolic of summer than sitting in an Adirondackchair, sipping a cool, sweating glass of lemonade? Depending on how you infuse it, you may not want to leave your chair. Because lemonade has such a distinct sour/tangy taste, it masks the taste of CBD drops and pairs well with THC fruit-flavored beverages, too.

INGREDIENTS

2 cups water

2 cups sugar

5 pounds fresh lemons

Liquid CBD (drops) or commercially produced THC-infused fruit beverage (optional)

DIRECTIONS

Make a simple syrup: heat water in a saucepan over medium heat. Stir in sugar. Keep cooking and stir occasionally until the liquid looks clear.

Now, begin juicing lemons and continue until you have 2 cups of lemon juice.

Combine the simple syrup with the lemon juice and add water and ice to taste.

Put a few of the juiced lemon halves in the pitcher for visual effect. You may even want to serve it in a mason jar, and by all means, find yourself an Adirondack chair to sit in.

Serves 4 to 6.

Note: This is not infused. It is just a great glass of happiness. If you want to infuse it, add liquid CBD drops or add some commercially produced THC-infused fruit beverage.

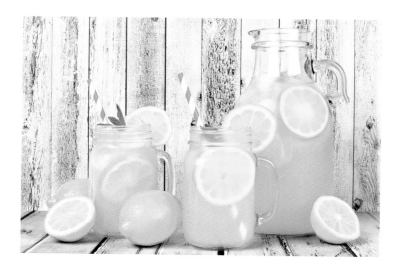

BANG BANG CUPCAKES
(Chocolate Cupcakes with Red Chili Pepper)

It may be an unlikely combination, but chocolate and chili work well together. The slight bitterness of the chocolate melds with the sugar and coconut, and then, bang, your taste buds are hit with some unexpected heat. A rich buttercream or slightly sour cream cheese frosting makes a perfect topping for this dramatic dessert.

INGREDIENTS

Batter:

½ cup flour

1 teaspoon baking powder

Pinch of salt

¼ cup sugar

⅓ cup cocoa or cacao

½ to 1 teaspoon red pepper flakes

3 tablespoons infused coconut oil, melted

¾ cup milk (or nut milk)

1 teaspoon vanilla

¼ teaspoon apple cider vinegar

1 can buttercream or cream cheese frosting or refer to frosting recipes on page 136

DIRECTIONS

Grease a muffin tin, or place liners in muffin tin wells. Preheat oven to 365°F.

In a large bowl, whisk: flour, baking powder, salt, sugar, cocoa or cacao, and ½ to 1 teaspoon red pepper flakes.

Create a well in the middle of the dry ingredients. Add melted infused coconut oil, milk (or nut milk), vanilla, and apple cider vinegar.

Beat the batter until all lumps disappear.

Fill 4 to 5 cupcake liners two-thirds full.

Bake for 20 minutes or until toothpick comes out clean.

Let them cool completely before frosting.

Serves 4 to 5.

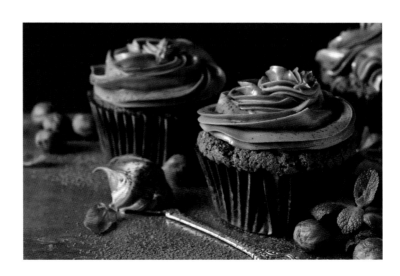

THUMBPRINT COOKIES

*"What should I put in the center of my thumbprint cookies?" is a
creative quandary to have. Traditionally, pieces of chocolate or a small
dollop of peanut butter or any fruit preserve works well. Whatever you decide,
these cookies are a little bite of heaven and don't take much time to make.*

INGREDIENTS

1¼ cups flour

Pinch of salt

⅓ cup sugar

2 tablespoons infused coconut oil, melted

2 tablespoons non-infused coconut oil, melted

½ teaspoon vanilla

¼ cup milk (or nut milk), room temperature

Peanut butter, jelly, or chocolate candies (or a combination)

DIRECTIONS

Preheat oven to 350°F and line a cookie sheet with parchment paper.

In a large bowl, whisk flour, salt, and sugar.

Add melted infused and non-infused coconut oil, vanilla, and milk or nut milk (at room temperature).

Mix and knead dough until smooth.

Pull 1-inch chunks off the dough ball. Roll chunks into spheres.

Place cookies on prepared baking sheet and press the center with your thumb.

Fill divot with peanut butter, jelly, chocolate candy, or other sweet treat.

Bake 15 to 20 minutes, until golden.

Serves 6.

BUTTERCREAM AND CREAM CHEESE FROSTING

INGREDIENTS

½ cup unsalted butter, softened

2 cups confectioners' sugar, sifted

1½ teaspoons vanilla

2 tablespoons milk or nut milk

Food coloring (optional)

DIRECTIONS

Using a hand mixer (or by hand) beat butter slowly until smooth. Add confectioners' sugar a little at a time until it's folded in. Mix in vanilla. Pour in milk or nut milk and beat for several more minutes until smooth and spreadable. If using food coloring, add a drop at a time until you see desired color.

Makes enough frosting for 8 to 12 cupcakes or 1 cake.

For cream cheese variation, beat an 8-ounce block of cream cheese before adding the butter and following the rest of the recipe. Omit milk.

TAHINI MAPLE SUGAR COOKIES

If you are looking for cookies with unique levels of flavor, you have found the right recipe. You may recognize tahini as an ingredient in hummus and in this recipe it shares the spotlight with maple syrup, coconut, and vanilla. The result is a distinct, pleasing bite every time.

INGREDIENTS

1 cup flour

1/2 teaspoon baking powder

1/4 teaspoon salt

1/4 cup tahini

2 tablespoons infused coconut oil, room temperature

2 tablespoons non-infused coconut oil, room temperature

1/2 cup sugar

1/2 teaspoon vanilla

1/2 cup maple syrup

DIRECTIONS

Line cookie sheet with parchment paper. Preheat oven to 375°F.

In a medium bowl, whisk flour, baking powder, and salt.

In a large bowl, combine tahini, infused and non-infused coconut oil, sugar, vanilla, and maple syrup.

Mix together dry and wet ingredients.

Scoop 2-inch balls onto prepared cookie sheet.

Press tops flat with a fork and sprinkle with sugar.

Bake 12 to 15 minutes, until lightly golden.

Serves 6.

BROWNIE BITES

No cannabis recipe section would be complete without an infused brownie recipe.
It's the ultimate way to happily wrap up a meal with a sweet chocolate rich bite.

INGREDIENTS

¾ cup sugar

¾ tablespoon baking powder

¼ teaspoon salt

½ cup cocoa or cacao

8 teaspoons
  infused butter, melted

⅓ cup non-infused
  coconut oil, melted

2 eggs

1 tablespoon vanilla

¾ cup flour

⅓ cup walnuts or chocolate
  chips (optional)

DIRECTIONS

Grease 8 wells of a muffin tin, or fill with cupcake liners. Preheat oven to 350°F. In a large bowl, whisk sugar, baking powder, salt, and cocoa or cacao. Then mix in melted infused butter, coconut oil, eggs, and vanilla. Fold in the flour and, if desired, walnuts or chocolate chips.

Fill muffin tins or cupcake liners three-quarters full.

Bake 18 to 24 minutes. Take out of oven when batter begins to pull away from the sides and when they spring back when lightly poked. Cool until slightly warm.

Serves 8.

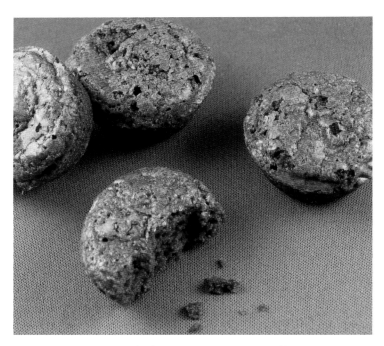

This recipe and several others appear courtesy of home cannacook Corinne Tobias. Visit her at wakeandbake.co.

KEY LIME (OH MY) HIGH PIE

As I was learning to bake, this was one of the first pies I mastered. If desired, you can substitute animal crackers or ginger snaps for the crust. As David Mamet said, "We must have a pie. Stress cannot exist in the presence of a pie." I totally agree.

INGREDIENTS

Crust:

2 cups graham cracker crumbs

3 tablespoons non-infused butter

3 tablespoons infused butter

½ cup sugar

Filling:

8-ounce can condensed milk

3 eggs

1¼ cups key lime juice

½ cup plain yogurt or sour cream

Lime zest (or very thinly sliced lime pieces) for decoration

DIRECTIONS

Heat oven to 350°F.

In a large bowl, mix crust ingredients. Press with your fingers and a fork into a 9-inch pie pan.

Bake for 5 minutes. Let cool while you prepare the filling.

For the filling, whisk ingredients until smooth.

Fill the pie pan and return to the oven for another 5 to 7 minutes. Let the pie cool and, if possible, let chill for another 2 hours.

Before serving, sprinkle with lime zest or decorate with thin lime slices.

Serves 8.

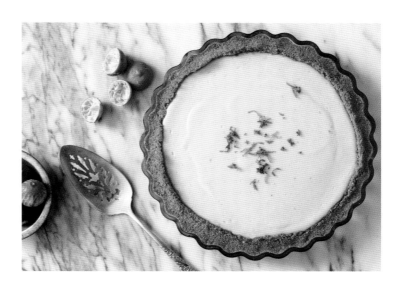

Chapter 7

AN INFUSED DINNER PARTY:
Two Proven Approaches

Now that you are knowledgeable about cannabis, familiar with how to infuse butters and oils with cannabis, and practiced in creating delicious recipes using those infusions, you may be wondering how you can introduce curious friends to the brave new world of cannabis. This desire to share the experience with others in a safe and fun way is what led me to create the dinner party branch of Our Community Harvest. Cannabis-infused dinner parties are a fantastic way to expose your interested friends to the delights of cannabis. Keep reading for information on how to throw a non-intimidating party, whether your guests are novices or experienced.

Setting the Stage for a Successful Party

First, you need to prepare the THC oil or butter infusion, making sure to correctly calculate the dosage of 1 tablespoon and 1 teaspoon. We have found that THC (sativa dominant) infused olive oil works very well for appetizers, side dishes, and entrées, and that infused coconut oil (indica dominant) works well for desserts and baked goods. If you are limited to one infusion, you may want to use infused butter (a balanced sativa/indica infusion) for all of your infused dishes,

but honestly, it is better if you have separate sativa and indica infusions.

When you send out invitations for your party, make sure that anyone who is planning on trying cannabis has a designated driver lined up.

The First Approach— Microdosing for Less- Experienced Guests

Before the party, plan a simple menu featuring dishes you have made before (whether they are from the previous chapter or from your own repertoire) that can be easily individually infused; essentially, you will be drizzling precisely calculated amounts of oil over a simple dish. Because you are infusing your dishes, you don't want to add a layer of complexity by making new dishes.

As your guests arrive, have a few non-infused appetizers and non-alcoholic drinks ready to go. Let them know that you'll talk about what will happen over the course of the evening once everyone arrives, and reassure them that the appetizers and drinks they are enjoying are neither infused nor alcoholic. Above all, you want your guests to feel comfortable and confident that you know what you are doing. As your guests mill around and talk, you'll feel the excitement building into an attentive audience.

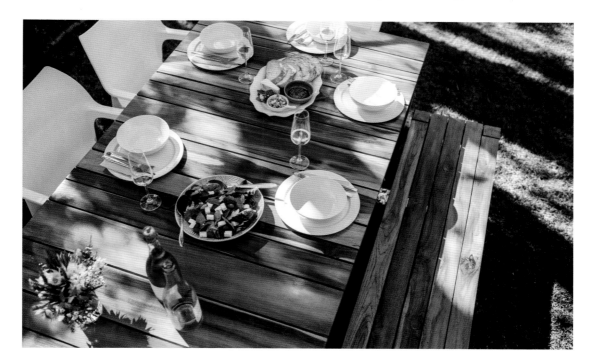

Overview of the Evening

Once everyone arrives, give an overview of the evening. Let your guests know that none of the dishes will be infused unless the guest requests an infusion, and you will give them guidance as to how much they may want to try. Take a moment to let them know how carefully you created the oil and how you calculated the potency; try to keep this as simple as possible because it can get too technical very easily. Explain that each guest can customize his or her experience by microdosing non-infused dishes with cannabis oil as they prefer.

Point out that the infused oil features a sativa-dominant oil, which will increase one's appetite and sense of well-being; guests may feel laughter coming on, and the high is likely to be felt primarily in the head, but may be present in the body as well. The infused dessert is indica- and CBD-dominant, so your guests will arrive home content and ready for a great night's sleep.

One thing to keep in mind is that some of your guests may start feeling impatient if they don't feel effects after 45 minutes or an hour. I remember one of my friends at an infused dinner party after an hour saying, "I don't think it's working." But I encouraged him to be patient. Sure enough, after another 15 minutes, he said, "I feel like someone just put a blanket on me and I can tell that I'm going to be really talkative." And he was talkative, by the way. The takeaway here is that you should remind your guests to go "Low and Slow"; try a low dose, take your time, and don't enhance your experience by smoking or vaping cannabis or by drinking alcohol. The "extra" smoke and liquor will skew the infusion experience and you may not be able to figure out a dose you are comfortable with. Of course, the remarkable thing about edibles is that you can eat edibles the very next day if you want to. So, you'll figure out a comfortable dose if you are patient.

Drinks

We like to greet the guests with an uninfused lemonade (see page 134). However, there are a few options for infused beverages:

- If you are in California, you can try No Label wine, which is infused with cannabis
- The Green Drink (page 132)
- Strava Craft Coffee (infused with CBD, so it makes a great companion with or after dessert)

Appetizers

Relay the fact that the party will start with appetizers infused upon request, and that effects may be felt 30 minutes up to 2 hours after consuming the appetizer. Here are a couple popular appetizers we find work well with a microdosing format.

- Mozzarella, Tomato, and Basil Bite (page 121)
- Bruschetta (page 121)
- Scallops (page 121)
- Shrimp (page 121)
- Garlic and Goat Cheese Toast (page 121)

After the appetizers have been served, remind your guests that it will take a while for the effects to start, and also remind them that when you

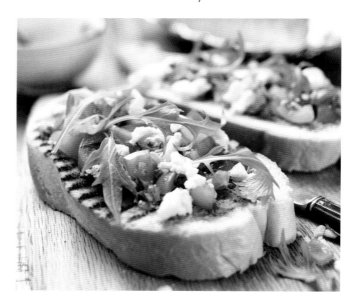

eat edibles, the effects last much longer. In contrast to smoking cannabis, where effects are felt in about 5 minutes and last about 2 hours, edibles won't hit for at least half an hour up to 2 hours and effects can last from 4 to 8 hours. This is one of the reasons that if you dose edibles correctly, you are likely to have deep, glorious, non-interrupted sleep.

Side Dishes

At this point, take a moment to check in with your guests to see how they are feeling. More adventurous guests may want to increase their dose, and they can do so with an infused side dish.

Remind your guests that if they are not feeling anything yet or only a mild buzz, that they may want to try another drizzle on their side dish; if they choose the additional infusion, it is almost certain that they will feel something by dessert. For example, if a diner ate a microdosed appetizer (at 2.5 mg) and then waited until the main course and had another microdose (2.5 mg) on a side dish, it is highly likely that they will feel some effects by dessert. Remember the goal is to find out what the smallest dose is that works for each individual.

Here are some great side dishes that are easy to microdose:

* Mixed Green Salad (page 123)
* Baby Spinach Salad with Strawberries and Walnuts (page 122)
* Three Bean Salad (page 122)
* Gazpacho (page 123)
* Roasted Seasonal Vegetables (page 123)

Entrée

Now we move on to the entrée portion of the meal. Because microdosing is the method in use here, you should prepare a non-infused dish.

Here are some popular entrées from our recipe chapter, but keep in mind to use only non-infused oils and butters for the novice party. Guests can microdose as needed.

* Soy Marinated Chicken Thighs with Lemon Zest (page 128)
* Udon Noodles with Veggies in Veggie Broth (page 127)
* Vegetable Lasagna (page 129)
* Skirt Steak Drizzled with Chimichurri Sauce (page 130)
* Fish in Parchment Paper on a Bed of White Beans, Arugula, Cherry Tomatoes, Garlic, and Sausage (page 131)

Now that the main course is on the table and guests are eating, you will start to see and hear the party kick into party mode. You'll know that the party is going well when you start hearing laughter and the noise level

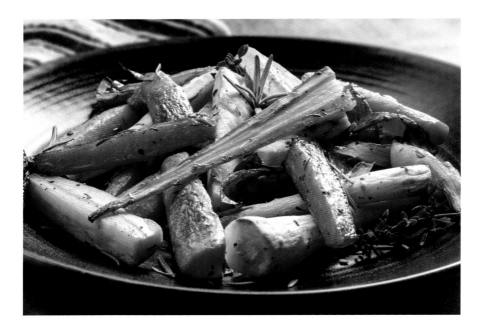

increases. This also gives you a chance to glance over the partygoers to see if it looks like anyone is uncomfortable, though using the microdose approach mitigates the chance of this happening. If it does, refer to page 88, where we talk about what to do if you have an uncomfortable high.

Dessert

The classic cannabis dessert is brownies and, because I have never met anyone who dislikes a brownie, that's what I would suggest serving. Here are a couple of terrific tips I've learned about serving brownies at an infused party. First, I once made the mistake of making a tray of brownies and cal-culated that each piece—which was a respectable 3" x 3"—had an infusion of 10 mg. So, if someone wanted a smaller dose such as 5 mg, they would have to cut the brownie in half. And if they wanted a 2.5 mg dose, they could have a quarter of a brownie. I bet you know where this is going—no one wants half a brownie and they definitely don't want a quarter of a brownie! The solution is to make a traditional pan of brownies that are not infused so everyone can have a proper dessert. The indica infusion arrives in the form of Brownie Bites, which are small infused brownies (see page 138).

Once the indica-infused dessert is served (which will start to relax your guests and will signal to the body that it's time to rest), let your guests know that ideally, they should be on their way home within about half an hour, so they can enjoy the restful experience in the comfort of their home. You may also want to suggest that they write down some impressions and details of the night, so they can track their successful consumption. For example, they should note what dose they took, when they began to feel effects, and describe the effects. Upon waking, they should record what happened when they got home, how they slept, and any lingering effects they felt. In this way, they will know what is right for their body and will learn how to repeat a successful experience.

It bears repeating that guests who are high should not be driving, so arrange rides and designated drivers before the event.

Second Approach— Fully Infused Dishes for Experienced Users

If you are hosting an infused dinner party where your guests are comfortable and familiar with cannabis—that is, they are regular or semi-regular users—here is another dinner party approach. In general, the pace is similar to the microdose dinner party, but instead of using the drizzle technique,

entire infused dishes are created. You can use a recipe from this book (see chapter 6), or infuse your favorite recipe by simply replacing traditional oil with infused oil.

◆ As your guests gather, we like to have a non-infused, fun beverage to serve them to set the mood. As they enjoy their drink and a small non-infused appetizer, the flow of the party is explained. We are big fans of lemonade served in a large mason jar so that's what we suggest here (see page 134).

◆ When everyone arrives, let them know that infused dishes will be clearly marked and that non-infused dishes will be available with each course as well.

◆ When creating infused dishes, you need to calculate at what level the entire dish is infused. Then, you determine how much a guest would eat when they consume a normal portion. In other words, if you served infused hummus (page 119), you would designate on a label what the total infusion is in the dish, and then indicate how potent 1 table-spoon is—which is about how much someone would eat as a usual portion—by saying it contains x amount of THC. In this way, a guest can decide how much they want to eat to achieve their desired

Profile

CANNABIS ON THE MENU

SHATTA MEJIA, *Home Cannacook and Cannabis Enthusiast*

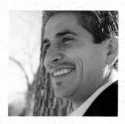

When I was in 6th grade, I started to have a hard time with what I was being fed; I'm sure the food was just like any other large, working-class Mexican family, but for some reason, my stomach frequently rejected my diet. I got cramps consistently in middle school and the beginning of freshman year. I met a friend in February of that year who was a vegetarian—more because of the Grateful Dead than any health concerns. After cooking with him a few times, I decided to go home and tell my family I was going vegetarian. I did, and for the next 4 years, I did not eat red meat, pork, or poultry. I still ate fish, but not often. This is where I gained a love of food and an appreciation for the time it takes to cook well.

As a musician, I started traveling the country, then the world, when I was 20; this coincided with the decision to eat anything and everything my hosts offered and to cook what I learned to enjoy eating. There was no place I was not allowed to venture in my culinary trails; I started with fusion dishes very early and learned from experienced cooks every chance I got.

I now travel around the country cooking infused dinners using local marijuana and ingredients; I cook affordable, working-class food with updated techniques and ingredients. Being a lifelong marijuana smoker has allowed me to understand the best techniques to infuse food. Every time I create a new fusion dish, I make sure I know what dosage I would include for each portion. After trying various butters and oils, I prefer Indian ghee from any international market for infusing dishes that call for butter or oil.

effect. To review what was taught earlier on dosing, here is an example. If you started with 7 grams (1/4 ounce) of 15% THC flower/bud and made 16 ounces (2 cups) of infused olive oil, your potency would be 25 mg THC per tablespoon or 8 mg per teaspoon. So, if you used 2 tablespoons of infused oil in your hummus, there would be a total of 50 mg of THC in the dish. If the dish yielded 10 servings, each serving is 5 mg of THC. Mark your infused dish with dosage information—such as "This hummus contains 5 mg of THC per serving." Don't forget to have non-infused options on hand.

- Remind diners that effects will take 30 minutes up to 2 hours to kick in and explain how edibles are different than smoking; remind them that if they smoke or drink alcohol during an infused dinner that effects will be magnified.

- Let your dinner guests know that the infused appetizers, side dishes, and entrées are all infused with a sativa strain, which is associated with energy, creativity, and laughter.

- Even though you are serving experienced cannabis users, let them know that it is recommended that they start with an infused appetizer and see how they feel before possi-

bly eating an infused side dish and/or entrée.

- Before you serve an infused entrée and side dishes, your experienced audience may want to smoke a bit, so make sure to have a designated smoking area away from the rest of the party if possible, as some diners don't like smoke at all. When your diners who smoke rejoin the party, they will most likely be high; when the appetizer is felt, the party will move into high gear. It also bears repeating that if you serve alcohol, serve it in moderation because it will react with the cannabis. So, guests may want to cut their normal alcohol consumption in half and should stay hydrated. You want this to be a pleasurable experience, and one way to ruin the experience is to consume too much alcohol and cannabis.

- Inform your guests that the dessert is infused with an indica strain, which is associated with relaxation, pain relief, and sleep—the goal is to have a high energy, fun party and then when dessert hits, it puts guests in the mood to relax.

- Reassure your guests that if they get too high, they should let you know; when this happens, they should hydrate and, if desired, take

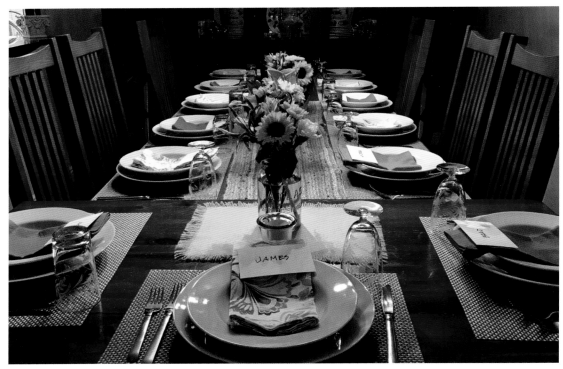

Hosting an infused dinner party is a great way to introduce the benefits of cannabis to your friends.

CBD drops or gum, which will help them level out.

- Finally, make sure that your guests have a safe ride home or a designated driver.
- At the end of the evening, give guests a "to go" infused gift, which may be a small baked good, some candy, or some flavored nuts. It's a nice touch at the end of the evening.

- Always include plenty of non-infused food options for your guests.
- Finally, if you are the main host and cook for an infused dinner, you probably shouldn't partake. I know, that doesn't sound like much fun! But that way you can dose correctly and ensure your guests are safe and have an enjoyable experience. And of course, as you teach guests to infuse, they'll certainly return the favor at some point.

Entertaining Tips

To be prepared for your infused cannabis party, here are a few things you can infuse or do in advance; we will also cover some general entertaining tips:

Examples of things you can do ahead include prepping vegetables and keeping them in the fridge until you are ready to use them. You can also make some pizza dough, muffin batter, or pie dough to keep them on hand as well. These are just a few simple examples, and of course there are many more items you can prep ahead; it all depends on the type of appetizers, dinner, and dessert you want to serve.

The key is to make a menu ahead of time, figure out how many portions you have to make, and plan to prep or make as many things in advance as is reasonable. Especially when infusing for the first time, plan on making simple dishes that you have mastered. I would also increase the amount of food I normally serve, as I find guests tend to consume a bit more than usual—probably because of the munchies!

And to give yourself a bit of a break, think about recruiting a trusted friend to bring some non-infused appetizers or a dessert. For emergencies, you'll also want to have items on hand such as chips and dip, glazed nuts, cheese and crackers, spiced olives, pre-made salad, croutons, and vanilla ice cream.

Other things to consider are:

- Whether you want to have assigned seating.
- What type of music, if any, that you will supply—on OurCommunityHarvest.com we have a cannabis music playlist (feel free to make suggestions of songs we should add).
- If possible, set the table in advance.
- Plan to clean as you go.
- Have an emergency backup plan in case something happens; I personally almost always have a vegetarian lasagna in the freezer as back up.
- Above all, have fun, keep the food simple and fresh—especially for your first infused meal—and if you plan and prep ahead, things will go smoothly.
- Good luck!

Chapter 8
LOOKING FORWARD

As we enter a period of increased cannabis legalization and as more citizens consider the place of cannabis in their lives, we will encounter several key obstacles and challenges that must be addressed. Let's take a brief look at the biggest misunderstandings about cannabis and how to take action.

- Is cannabis addictive?
- Is cannabis a gateway drug?
- What do we do about kids and cannabis (and pets)?
- How do we curb and test for driving while high?
- What can we do regarding banking and the security of large amounts of cash resulting from the cannabis industry?

Is Cannabis Addictive?

The question "Is cannabis addictive?" is one of the most searched questions on Google. From speaking with many people who posed this question, I noticed they were usually motivated by a few common factors. First, some were motivated by self-interest, as they began to consider whether they could or should use cannabis for pain relief, relaxation, or any number of conditions. Remember that for some people, this is a huge leap of faith. They may have grown up as D.A.R.E. kids (Drug and Alcohol Resistance Ed-

ucation courses are still being offered in a number of schools and many kids who come out of the program are educated to fear cannabis and other substances), or perhaps they are older and grew up in a time of prohibition and stereotypes and are reluctant to consider cannabis. But as we all know, once a real health concern appears on your doorstep, you look to advice, information, and remedies that you may have easily dismissed before. I have also found that once someone close to you uses cannabis for health successfully—whether in the form of CBD, THC, or a combination—that it becomes "okay" to investigate.

When looking at whether cannabis is addictive, I think one of the most useful ways to look at it is to compare "cannabis addiction"—which is more like cannabis dependence or a cannabis habit—to other forms of addiction. For example, did you wake up today and have a cup of coffee or two? Did you smoke a cigarette? Or at about 6 pm last night did you have a glass of wine? All of these activities could be looked at as dependencies, habits, or addictions. Cannabis is similar; users may pursue a pattern of behavior where they like to consume cannabis at certain times of the day because it causes certain results. Similar to coffee, if a habitual cannabis user

Profile

COMMON-SENSE, COMMUNITY-BASED APPROACH

JOE DISALVO, *Pitkin County (Aspen, CO) Sheriff*

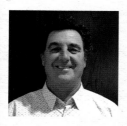

My experience with marijuana began in the mid-1970s growing up a few miles from New York City. The source was usually someone's older brother who "scored" and was willing to make a quick buck selling low-grade weed and seed. The exchange usually took place in the high school parking lot, where the fear of police and school administrators was high. Getting caught meant extreme consequences.

In 1980, I left New York for Aspen, Colorado. I was unprepared for the cannabis-friendly culture. Even then, drug use was seen as a personal choice, as long as your choice did not hurt or affect others negatively. Marijuana was prevalent and the police were "cool," as long as you made smart choices on where and when you consumed it. Police openly said marijuana was below jaywalking as a public safety risk. This attitude was refreshing to me and made sense. In fact, most skiers considered marijuana a performance-enhancing drug, as most still do. Riding a chairlift and smoking a joint was a regular and accepted occurrence, as long as you weren't stupid.

In 1985, I joined the Aspen Police Department as a patrol officer. As part of my training, I was told not to spend too much time on marijuana unless public users were flagrant and "not cool." A few years later, I joined the

Pitkin County Sheriff's Office; the sheriff, Bob Braudis, had the same philosophy regarding marijuana, which I shared throughout my career. I found out early that the war on drugs was a costly waste of time and resources.

In 2011, I was elected as the Pitkin County Sheriff. In November 2012, 3.6 million Coloradans voted on Amendment 64, a ballot initiative to legalize, sell, and regulate marijuana like alcohol. It passed with 55.3%; Colorado became the first state to legalize marijuana. The first retail sale was January 1, 2014. In the first year, 99 million dollars in legal marijuana was sold. The tax revenue was a windfall for the state and school infrastructure.

I'm often asked how legal marijuana has affected our town. The answer is, it hasn't, primarily because we have always had a cannabis-friendly culture. We've taken a responsible approach by educating locals and visitors alike, teaching buyers how to use responsibly, especially edibles. Aspen was one of the first cities to ban look-alike infused candy. If the product looked like a product that would be attractive to a child, our dispensaries volunteered not to sell it. Now look-alike products are banned from dispensaries statewide. I believe our community and state have done a model job of the responsible introduction of this product into Colorado. I believe our success is based on our past attitudes and historical experiences toward marijuana that were based in reality and not fear.

stops using for a while, they may feel more irritable and not as energetic or relaxed, or may have trouble sleeping, but any other physical or mental effects will be minor. That is, there is no "withdrawal" as you may be envisioning when an alcohol or drug addict stops using their substance. So, in the broadest sense, cannabis is only "addictive" to a minor population and this behavior can be controlled. If you suspect you may be prone to addiction but you want to try cannabis, you should start solely with CBD products. If you respond well, you can then try a bit of THC accompanied by CBD and see how you fare. In this way, you can find out what works best for your body. Above all, don't let fear stunt your journey.

Is Cannabis A Gateway Drug?

This is the argument and concern that is often voiced by cannabis opponents or those who have bought into the notion that cannabis is dangerous in any form. But simply, no, cannabis is not a gateway drug. When writing this book, I met so many people who had tried cannabis at one point in their life but never moved on to "harder drugs." It is not the case that if you use or like cannabis that you will crave more and move on to more potent substances.

The dependency argument gets conflated with correlation and not causation. In other words, people who initially try cannabis may be the same people who drink coffee or alcohol. But it doesn't mean that everyone who drinks coffee or alcohol will someday try cannabis and that cannabis users will eventually try harder drugs like meth or cocaine. Tens of thousands of people around you every day are using or have used cannabis, but will not or have not used stronger substances.

It is also helpful to look at treatment numbers. Nearly 60% of patients who are in rehabilitation for cannabis are there because their other choices were prison or probation, so it's easy to see why they chose rehabilitation. An additional 27% are under the age of 25 and are dealing with other substance issues, especially the abuse of alcohol and heroin.

Younger users may have some difficulty handling cannabis because their brains are not fully formed. Research suggests that you should be at least 25 before consuming cannabis (especially if it contains THC). Krista Lisdahl, director of brain imaging and neuropsychology at the University of Wisconsin, is quoted in Taryn Hillin's *Splinter* article, "Science Says Twenty-Somethings Probably Shouldn't

Profile

TALKING TO KIDS ABOUT CANNABIS

JESSIE GILL, *Marijuana Mommy*

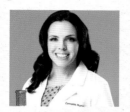

My first instinct after becoming a cannabis patient was to hide it from my kids. I didn't discuss the details of any other medication, so why should marijuana be different? Then, the D.A.R.E. education of my youth crept back to me. I wondered what would happen if my children came across the cannabis or overheard me discussing it. Would they assume it was illegal? Would they feel afraid for my well-being? Would they know it wasn't for them?

Kids are being sent contradictory messages from many directions; in the process, they're absorbing absurdly inaccurate data. Schools are still teaching propaganda-era information, comparing cannabis to heroin. Meanwhile, media and widespread legalization are demonstrating that cannabis is significantly safer. Parents need to be the authority. It's our responsibility to teach the benefits, risks, and expectations of healthy cannabis consumption.

Like all complicated topics (alcohol, sex, sexuality, addiction, racism), there are age-appropriate approaches. How we go about discussing it is less important than *if* we discuss it. Initiating the conversation is vital. A casual question is a great place to start: "What do you know about marijuana?" This can also be an excellent way to assess knowledge.

For younger children, explaining cannabis as a medicine or as a substance only for grown-ups is enough. As children age, they're better able to understand the complications of the law and the fight for social justice.

As parents prepare to discuss cannabis, they should ponder sharing information about personal use. Honesty is important; however, children should never be burdened with secrets of illegal activity. Additionally, kids who encounter cannabis regularly, for example, patients or family members of patients, should be prepared to face cannabis's negative stigma, as they're likely to run into it in school.

Legalization is rapidly approaching. Our children will encounter legal cannabis in their futures. If we don't provide our kids with accurate information, someone else will fill their minds with unhealthy myths and propaganda.

Smoke Weed," saying, "We have strong evidence that brain structure, especially in the prefrontal and parietal cortices, is still changing until age 25,' said Lisdahl. 'If we based it completely on science, I would recommend the age limit be 25." The message if you are under 25 is "Not Now"

Profile

CBD WORKS FOR PETS, TOO

DR. TIM SHU, *Veterinarian, Founder of VETCBD*

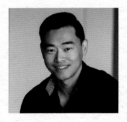

As a healthcare provider, it is my responsibility to provide clients with the best choices available for their pets' care. If cannabis has the ability to safely provide therapeutic benefit, I see it as my duty to explore those options. My research led me to realize the veterinary profession was far behind on the subject of cannabinoid therapy. The endocannabinoid system is present in humans and animals, and plays key roles in cognition, memory, appetite, pain, and immune system function; however, it was not taught in veterinary school, and certainly wasn't being discussed in practice.

In 2015, I left private practice and founded VETCBD to provide effective cannabinoid therapy to pets. Utilizing my clinical experiences, I formulated safe and effective cannabis products for pets. The products utilize full-spectrum CBD-rich cannabis and are non-psychoactive, meaning there is no "high." Fast-forward 3 years, and at the time of writing, we have been able to help tens of thousands of pets find relief from pain, anxiety, inflammation, nausea, seizures, and cognitive dysfunction. We have seen benefits in multiple species, including dogs, cats, rabbits, pigs, ferrets, rats, and horses.

The feedback and testimonials we have received from owners has been the most rewarding aspect and illustrates the life-changing capabilities of cannabinoid therapy. Here is just a single example:

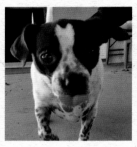

Jodie, a 6-year-old chihuahua diagnosed with epilepsy, had intractable seizures despite anti-seizure medication. She had upward of 20 seizures a day; her quality of life suffered to the point her owners were considering humane euthanasia to ease her suffering. Jodie's owner started her on our tincture and immediately saw a drastic decrease in seizure activity. Her quality of life returned and the owner reports they "have never seen Jodie so happy, playful, and above all, seizure free!"

Cannabinoid therapy is just as important in veterinary medicine as it is in human medicine. Like people, animals can benefit greatly from cannabinoid therapy when properly utilized, and as health professionals, we must advocate for further legalization and research of cannabinoid therapeutics if we are to act in our patients' and clients' best interests.

instead of "Not Ever." And again, this only applies to cannabis with THC and not CBD (Hillin 2015).

So, if you are considering cannabis for medicinal use, do not let the false gateway argument derail your journey. And if you are especially concerned, don't forget our friend, CBD.

What About Kids, Cannabis, and Pets?

As with other intoxicants and adult products, be responsible and keep cannabis away from kids and pets (and adults who do not want to partake). Label your products clearly, and keep them away from similar products. For example, if you have infused gummies, don't put them in a candy drawer or near other sweets. Consider purchasing a safe or a secure stash box and store in a safe location. Also, have the cannabis conversation with your kids—you will be glad you did.

Take special care that pets cannot access your products. Don't deliberately blow smoke in their faces or share edibles with them (especially chocolate, which can be toxic to pets). There are CBD products made especially for pets that you can administer under the care of a veterinarian. Be sure to pay attention to pet dosage requirements as well.

How Do We Curb and Test for Drivers Who Are High?

I'm sure we can all agree that we do not want drivers who are drunk or high to be on our roads.

But unlike drunk driving tests, there is currently no reliable test for driving while high. In fact, if a blood test is administered to a daily cannabis smoker even 30 days after their last joint, they would most likely test positive for cannabis. Cannabis and THC stay in one's system for quite a while, so there are many cases of false "driving while high" blood tests. And, blood tests are required when there is a fatal accident. This means that if a driver is definitely intoxicated, but also smoked a joint the day before, the test would say they were intoxicated and driving while high—even though they were not actively high. So, when statistics are compiled, this case could wrongly be attributed to "driving while high."

One possible solution is to develop a reliable test for active cannabis impairment. This could be funded by earmarking a small portion of tax revenue that results from cannabis sales to be used for the development of a reliable test. And of course, once one state develops a reliable test, it should be shared or licensed to other states in an effort to come up with a reasonable national standard. This would keep us all safer on the roads. Right now, there are several researchers who are testing cheek swabs, saliva tests, and more. Many expect major developments soon.

Another method of "testing" cannabis-impaired drivers is through police-administered observational tests. Police will look at a suspected driver's pupils and conduct agility and memory tests. Certain departments have trained their officers in observational techniques, but of course, these tests have human limitations and errors do occur.

If there is a small bright spot here, it is that generally, drivers who are high know that they are high and usually drive slower and are more careful. Peak impairment time is around 20 to 40 minutes after smoking. The best advice is to stay off the roads while impaired to keep us all safer.

What About Banking and the Use of and Security of Large Amounts of Cash?

You've probably read about the vast amounts of cash the cannabis industry is generating. In 2017, Colorado took in 1.5 billion dollars in legal cannabis sales, and this cash has to go somewhere.

Although California's recreational cannabis market was legally open as of January 1, 2018, implementation has been slow because of excessive taxes, the slow migration of medical patients to the recreational market, and a lack of testing services. Even so, BDS Analytics, a company that specializes in the cannabis market, predicted that California's cannabis industry will hit $2.9 billion in sales in 2018 and rise to nearly $5 billion in sales in 2019. As other states legalize recreational and/or medical cannabis, this cash explosion will continue.

The issue all comes down to banking. Because cannabis in all its forms is still federally illegal, banks that are subject to FDIC (Federal Deposit Insurance Corporation) rules do not knowingly get involved with money from the cannabis industry. Even companies who merely supply services and expertise to the cannabis industry or who only sell CBD and hemp oil are often denied banking services. So, this means that stories of dispensary owners carrying briefcases full of cash to legally pay their taxes are all too common. And as with other cash-based businesses, occasionally robberies and violence result.

One offshoot of the need to handle so much cash is the rise of the sale/rentals of ATM machines at dispensaries and the increase in the number of security companies who handle and protect cannabis cash. One intriguing possible solution is the creation of state-owned banks. Governor Phil Murphy of New Jersey has proposed the creation of a state bank to coincide with the launch of recreational cannabis. Murphy estimates that New Jersey will take in about 300 million dollars in tax revenue in the first year of legalization, which would largely go into the state bank. If New Jersey is successful, expect other states to follow, which may finally force the U.S. government to provide banking as well (or to miss out on billions in new and needed revenue).

Actionable Steps

As I was researching the many issues and attitudes surrounding cannabis, it became clear that we need to act on the following fronts:

- Reschedule cannabis from a Schedule I substance to a Schedule III substance.
- Push the FDA, NIDA, and DEA to allow responsible medical research for the most common conditions that medical cannabis is used for in many states.
- Legalize hemp production in all 50 states and slow our rate of import of hemp and hemp products from other countries.
- Lobby insurance companies (and Medicare and Medicaid) to recognize cannabis, CBD oil, and hemp oil as medicine and to pay for cannabis as they do for prescription drugs and opioids.
- Decriminalize the simple possession of cannabis in all 50 states and review cases of incarceration for first-time possession, with the goal to reduce the prison population and to train offenders for a place in society.

Now that you have a better understanding of the world of cannabis, you may be asking yourself, "What can I do to move the conversation forward?' or "What can I do to ensure that cannabis medicine gets to those who need it?" As with many things, education, research, and political action all contribute to move our society forward.

You can begin the education process by recommending some key Web sites, online courses, and cannabis books to friends and neighbors who would benefit from learning about cannabis. It is very likely that you will find a more welcoming audience than you expect. Start by emphasizing the natural medical benefits of cannabis—as opposed to opiates—and explaining the non-high effects of CBD. You can also make the case that the use of recreational cannabis should be left to the discretion of a responsible adult and that it is less destructive—and even more beneficial—than alcohol. Other factors to emphasize are the tax income from legalization, savings from freeing up law enforcement resources, and lives saved because fewer people would go to prison.

Reschedule and Research

The next major step to move the acceptance of cannabis forward is to promote rescheduling and research. The U.S. has some of the best researchers in the world, and it is a huge missed opportunity for us to overlook cannabis as a major type of research. The vast amount of anecdotal evidence that we have cannot be overlooked anymore. We could even start small, with research focusing on the medical conditions outlined by many individual states as benefiting from cannabis treatment.

To begin research, we need to support changes at three governmental agencies, namely the FDA, the DEA, and NIDA. However, the initial and largest stumbling block is the federal classification of cannabis as a Schedule I drug. A Schedule I drug, you may recall, is a drug that has no accepted medical benefits, like heroin. To change this classification, we need to support legislation, such as the recent bills put forth by Florida congressmen Matt Gaetz and Darren Soto, which called for the rescheduling of cannabis from Schedule I to Schedule III. This move would allow for the acknowledgement of cannabis' legitimate medical value and further support for access to medical marijuana. If we are successful in changing cannabis' classification from a Schedule I drug, several organizations have made it their mission to support cannabis research and much progress could soon be made. A couple of these organizations with good reputations are NORML, Project CBD, and the Marijuana Policy Project.

Let's Bring Hemp Back to Prominence

As you have discovered, hemp is an innocent bystander in the war against cannabis. Do we have a single good reason why hemp should not be grown in all 50 states? You will recall that it is useful plant and fiber and has had a long successful history in the U.S. Hemp can be used to create more than 25,000 useful products, is relatively fast growing, is pest resistant, and is a good replacement crop for tobacco and more. In addition, we already import hemp from other countries and have been doing so for decades. Isn't it time to make hemp an important part of our economy again? To do so, let's support hemp growth and research via the National Hemp Association and others. The National Conference of State Legislatures has even joined together to create a comprehensive informational Web site that provides insight into the hemp legalization movement. In addition, many states have their own active lobbying organizations.

Lobby the Insurance Companies

Until cannabis is rescheduled, insurance companies will not be allowed to pay for cannabis as medicine. I know of several cases where a fixed-income patient would prefer to take CBD or other forms of cannabis versus prescription drugs and opioids, but their insurance company will only pay for the latter. So, these fixed-income patients are trapped into using prescription drugs that are paid for. And in a further irony, some of these patients are prescribed Marinol—and insurance companies pay for this drug—which is a synthetic form of can-

nabis! One bright international note is that Germany is exploring the possibility of insurance companies being required to pay for cannabis when it is prescribed. Perhaps this international action will demonstrate that cannabis should finally be treated like other effective medications and will show it is cost effective.

One additional interesting debate and development is that it appears some patients addicted to opioids (and other drugs) can be successfully transitioned to simply using cannabis. This may appeal to insurance companies because their payouts would be smaller, and they would be helping patients. Some would argue that you are trading "one drug for another," but keep in mind that cannabis does not have the side effects that opioids and other drugs do, and that there is a real opportunity to successfully manage one's cannabis use. Because there are so many strains and products available, a physician could help tailor the cannabis experience to move a patient away from opioids. Or at a minimum, cannabis could be used in conjunction with fewer drugs. This debate will no doubt heat up as we take on the U.S. opioid epidemic and as more research about cannabis becomes available.

Decriminalize in All 50 States and Free First-Time Offenders

Cory Booker, a New Jersey congressman, proposed the Marijuana Justice Act of 2017. Booker's bill would decriminalize cannabis on the federal level. In addition, Booker's proposal would seek to address reparations related to racially disproportionate enforcement of marijuana laws, as well as expunging convictions for marijuana use or

Profile

DECIDING TO GET A MEDICAL CANNABIS CARD

ROBERT MARTINEZ, *Cannabis Medical Patient and Researcher*

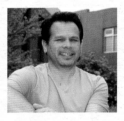

I decided to obtain a card both as a qualified patient, and to be afforded legal protection under my state's medical marijuana laws. The decision was not an easy one, considering there were many factors that I thought could upset my life. These included my professional goals, challenging the perception of who I was amongst family and friends, and a long-term desire to engage in the legal culture knowing for years of cannabis' medical benefits. While it took about a year to finally decide to move forward, I felt a real weight lifted and discovered a doorway to a world I thought I already understood.

I began investigating the options to deal with my medical needs, reading everything I could find. Thankfully, I was faced with multiple constructive avenues, all of which provided physical relief that complemented my busy professional and personal life. Best of all, I could maintain my beliefs with products that were all natural, and tailor prescriptions to fit my situations (working without a high using CBD-dominant products versus a light to moderate high during personal time). After identifying a few workable strains, I wondered why a country like the U.S. has prohibited this natural and affordable medicine. The answer to that, I found out, is a sordid story. I now share my research-based knowledge through teaching moments with family and friends to help educate others.

My final thought: Do not be afraid to engage in making prescriptive medical decisions for yourself versus the programmed manufactured choices. At least in New Mexico, if you want a card, there are a few options in your state to obtain one for anywhere from $50 to $200. Most doctors advertise MMJ cards openly in local newspapers and Web site searches. Be prepared to wait for the state to process your application over a 2 to 6 week period.

DID YOU KNOW?

Although the U.S. government considers cannabis to be a Schedule I substance, the Department of Health and Human Services filed a patent in 1998 that was approved in 2003 for cannabis as an antioxidant and neuroprotectant. It is patent number 6630507, and this hypocrisy has been highlighted widely in social media via a "talk to the hand campaign," whereby citizens have written the number 6630507 on their hand and submitted photos.

Here is the wording for the patent from the U.S. Patent Office:

"Cannabinoids have been found to have antioxidant properties, unrelated to NMDA receptor antagonism. This newfound property makes cannabinoids useful in the treatment and prophylaxis of wide variety of oxidation associated diseases, such as ischemic, age-related, inflammatory and autoimmune diseases. The cannabinoids are found to have particular application as neuroprotectants, for example in limiting neurological damage following ischemic insults, such as stroke and trauma, or in the treatment of neurodegenerative diseases, such as Alzheimer's disease, Parkinson's disease and HIV dementia. Nonpsychoactive cannabinoids, such as cannabidiol, are particularly advantageous to use because they avoid toxicity that is encountered with psychoactive cannabinoids at high doses useful in the method of the present invention. A particular disclosed class of cannabinoids useful as neuroprotective antioxidants is formula (I) wherein the R group is independently selected from the group consisting of H, CH_3, and $COCH_3$."

possession in an effort to perform restorative justice. This is just one example of the changing attitudes across the country. Part of the reason that Booker suggested this major change is to acknowledge that we have had a failed "War on Drugs" and that cannabis charges and arrests unfairly target people of color. Especially in the case of simple possession, thousands of minorities have been unfairly incarcerated at an enormous cost to their own lives, their families, their communities, and society overall. Given that medical and recreational use is booming across the nation and we are beginning to see the medical benefits and little harm that cannabis causes, it is the right time to decriminalize and to release first-time offenders through acts of restorative justice.

One key organization that is promoting cannabis change regarding policy and action is the Marijuana Policy Project (mpp.org). Their Web site contains a useful state-by-state guide and even includes contact information for your local representatives, governors, and more. I would encourage you to follow and support them if you are interested in real change. They make it so simple by providing letter templates, talking points, and specific information about cannabis issues affecting your community.

CANNABIS QUICK REVIEW: 70 IMPORTANT TAKEAWAYS

I bet you are surprised by the amount of information and, sometimes, the subtlety that exists in the cannabis world. To give you a broad overview, we've distilled the cannabis landscape into 70 quick, readable bullet points. Use this information to start informed conversations and to impress your friends and neighbors with your cannabis knowledge.

1. There are three main types of cannabis: sativa, indica, and hybrids.

2. Indica plants grow short and bushy; this strain is associated with relaxation and sleep.

3. Sativa plants grow tall and skinny; this strain is associated with energy and creativity.

4. Hybrid strains combine the best of both sativa and indica strains.

5. Ruderalis is another lesser-known member of the cannabis family; it can be CBD-rich and primarily grows in eastern Europe and Russia.

6. Hemp is a major source of fiber and is used to make thousands of different products from clothes to rope to beauty products.

7. Hemp was a very important crop for early colonists in America.

8. Between 1850 and 1937, cannabis was recognized for its positive medicinal qualities in the U.S.; several large pharmaceutical companies offered tinctures or drops for medical use.

9. The Marijuana Tax Act of 1937, fueled by anti-immigrant sentiments, signaled the beginning of criminalization of cannabis.

10. Hemp production in any capacity is allowed in 40 states.

11. Medical marijuana is legal in 30 states, Washington D.C., Puerto Rico, and Guam.

12. Recreational cannabis for adults 21 and over is now legal in Alaska, California, Colorado, Maine, Massachusetts, Nevada, Oregon, Vermont, Washington, and Washington D.C. and is soon expected to be legal in New Jersey and New Hampshire

(via the legislature rather than popular vote).

13. Michigan has collected enough votes to put the legalization of recreational cannabis on the ballot in 2018.

14. There are hundreds of slang terms for cannabis!

15. Uruguay was the first country in the world to completely legalize cannabis for adults.

16. Canada became the second with the official roll-out day on 10/17/18—Weed Wednesday.

17. There are new international developments in cannabis happening every day.

18. Arizona, Hawaii, Maine, Michigan, Nevada, New Hampshire, Pennsylvania, and Rhode Island all recognize medical marijuana cards from different states.

19. CBD, or cannabidiol, is a primary compound found in cannabis plants. It has analgesic, anti-inflammatory, and anti-anxiety properties that occur without making the user high.

20. CBD has been found effective in mitigating concussions if taken within four hours of trauma.

21. THC (tetrahydrocannabinol) is the chemical compound in cannabis that will give you a euphoric high.

22. Your body has an endocannabinoid system (ECS), which is a network of receptors and nerves; both THC and CBD adhere to the receptors or slow the breakdown of enzymes (though the receptors for THC and CBD are in different parts of the body) to provide benefits.

23. It is important to consult with your doctor about utilizing medical cannabis; ask plenty of questions!

24. There are strains that are CBD heavy for users who want to experience the medical benefits of cannabis without getting high.

25. Use a cannabis journal, especially as a beginner. It will help you keep track of your experiences and find what works best for you.

26. THC potency can be low (0% to 10%), medium (10% to 15%), or high (any greater than 15%).

27. Israeli scientist Raphael Mechoulam is fondly called the Grandfather of Cannabis; he was the first person to isolate THC.

28. Hemp is a great source of CBD, and hemp oil is often used in CBD products such as salves, gum, vapes, and tinctures.

29. Terpenes are the oils in cannabis that give it a distinctive smell.

30. Flavonoids are the aromatic molecules that contribute to the taste of cannabis.

31. If it's your first time visiting a dispensary, do research online and talk to your friends and your doctor about what to expect.

32. Always bring your ID, medical card, and cash to a dispensary.

33. Medical patients often pay less for cannabis products.

34. Ask the budtenders questions; they're there to help!

35. Depending on the state, some dispensaries offer delivery services.

36. Cannabis can be grown naturally outdoors, in a greenhouse, or indoors with artificial lights.

37. Home-growing a single plant isn't too difficult; simply acquire a good light and follow the instructions that are outlined on pages 50 and 51.

38. Only female cannabis plants produce the flower that cannabis enthusiasts consume.

39. Growers discard male plants as soon as possible so they don't pollinate the female plants.

40. Before partaking in cannabis, figure out what goal you have in mind.

41. Smoking is the most popular form of cannabis consumption.

42. Before smoking, the consumer should grind up the cannabis buds.

43. Joints are rolled with rolling papers and blunts are rolled with cigar wrappers.

44. Bowls are small glass or silicone pipes.

45. Bongs are larger glass or silicone pipes that use water.

46. Vaporizers are another method of consumption. Here, you inhale vapor instead of smoke.

47. Tinctures are cannabis-infused liquid drops; these are often used for medicinal purposes.

48. Edibles are cannabis-infused foods, ranging from stereotypical pot brownies to infused professional meals.

49. Topicals are cannabis-infused salves and ointments that are often CBD-based.

50. Suppositories are inserted in the rectum or vagina and deliver an impressive dose of medicine in a short time.

51. Advanced methods of consumption include cannabis concentrates such as dab, wax, and oil.

52. Hash is concentrated cannabis; a small piece looks like a piece of tar.

53. Kief is the potent "dust" that is left behind when you grind cannabis buds. It is often sprinkled on the top of bud in a joint or pipe for a more potent experience; makes wonderful infused oil, too.

54. If you have an uncomfortable high, sleep and hydration are the best ways to combat your experience.

55. Infused butters and oils (fats) are the basic building blocks of cooking with cannabis.

56. Consuming cannabis and alcohol simultaneously will magnify your experience.

57. Accurately dosing your edibles is key! Visit OurCommunityHarvest.com/calculator for a dosing calculator.

58. Store your infused butters and oils in airtight glass jars in a dark, cool place. Also, make sure to properly label them.

59. Infused butter can be frozen for several months if you need long-term storage.

60. Be sure to check for mold—which looks like wispy spider webs—on raw bud.

61. Early preparation and planning leads to a successful dinner party.

62. Make your infused oil and/or butter before any infused dinner party.

63. When your guests arrive, let them know what to expect for the evening and how the flow of the dinner party will work.

64. Remember that, unlike smoking cannabis, when you eat infused food, it may take from 30 minutes to 2 hours to feel the effects.

65. Correct dosing is vital when it comes to throwing dinner parties. Always go low and slow.

66. After consuming edibles, the effects may last 4 to 8 hours, so plan accordingly.

67. Be sure to offer non-infused courses in your dinner party.

68. Start with a sativa-infused appetizer, offer a regular entrée, and follow with an indica-infused dessert.

69. Another technique to use at a dinner party is called microdosing: each dish is infused with a small amount of cannabis—such as 2.5 milligrams.

70. As you continue your cannabis journey, remember to consult the annotated list of useful Web sites (page 172). Two strong advocacy sites are norml.org and mpp.org.

SELECTED READING & DOCUMENTARY LIST

Backes, Michael. 2014. **Cannabis Pharmacy: The Practical Guide to Medical Marijuana.** Elephant Book Company Limited.

Barcott, Bruce. 2015. **Weed the People: The Future of Legal Marijuana in America.** Time Books.

Casarett, David. 2015. **Stoned: A Doctor's Case for Medical Marijuana.** New York: Current.

Catalano, Jessica. 2012. **The Ganja Kitchen Cookbook.** Green Candy Press.

Dolce, Joe. 2016. **Brave New Weed: Adventures into the Uncharted World of Cannabis.** Harper Wave.

Dufton, Emily. 2017. **Grass Roots: The Rise and Fall and Rise of Marijuana in America.** Basic Books.

Graf, Nichole, Sherman, Micah, Stein, David, and Crain, Liz. 2017. **Grow Your Own: Understanding, Cultivating, and Enjoying Cannabis.** Tin House Books.

Klein, Zach. 2015. **The Scientist: Are We Missing Something?** Y. Klinik Productions.

Picillo, Ashley and Devine, Lauren. 2017. **Breaking the Grass Ceiling.** CreateSpace Independent Publishing Platform.

Pollan, Michael. 2009. **The Botany of Desire.** Kikim Media.

Rosenfeld, Irvin. 2011. **My Medicine: How I Convinced the U.S. Government to Provide My Marijuana and Helped Launch a National Movement.** Open Archive Press.

Tardiff, Joseph, ed. 2008. **Marijuana: Contemporary Issues Companion.** Greenhaven Press.

The Leafly Team. 2017. **The Leafly Guide to Cannabis.** Twelve.

Tobias, Corinne. 2017. **Dazed and Infused.** Wake and Bake Ventures Ltd.

Tobias, Corinne. 2013. **The Wake and Bake Cookbook,** Wake and Bake Publishing.

Wolf, Laurie and Parks, Melissa. 2015. **Herb.** Inkshares.

ANNOTATED WEB SITES

Our Community Harvest

Our Community Harvest is a
community for people who want to
learn about and contribute cannabis
knowledge. Online courses, in-person
seminars, and cooking demonstrations
are offered, as well as curated and
tested cannabis products—especially
CBD products—and noteworthy
information on the melding of
cannabis and food.
OurCommunityHarvest.com

Cannabis Now

This Web site and magazine's news
section addresses current events,
economics, legal topics, and politics
of cannabis, as well as cultivation,
edibles, medical marijuana topics, and
strains. Resources on the history of
cannabis, dispensary profiles, events,
and product reviews are also found.
CannabisNow.com

DOPE Magazine

If you live in Arizona, California,
Colorado, Nevada, Oregon, or
Washington, there is a version of
DOPE Magazine tailored to your
community. There is also a national
version. Their site covers news,
lifestyle, grow hints, legal and political
issues, and strain and product reviews.
As its name suggests, the publication
is a blend of a serious articles and a
more light-hearted approach to all
things cannabis related.
DopeMagazine.com

Future Cannabis Project

The Future Cannabis Project Web
site emphasizes coverage of four
main marijuana topics: health, policy,
business, and culture. It's a great site
for a quick overview of current events.
FutureCannabisProject.com

Laurie and MaryJane

This is the Web site of accomplished
cannabis chef Laurie Wolf. She runs
an award-winning edibles business in
Portland, Oregon. If you are fortunate
enough to live in Oregon, you can
purchase her precisely dosed oils,
butters, peanut butter, and edible
treats. Check out her recipes on her
blog, DontFearTheEdible.com, as well.
LaurieandMaryJane.com

Leafly

Leafly is particularly useful when it
comes to researching strains and
dispensaries. There are plenty of
lists, charts, reviews, and tips. If you
are researching strains, start with
peer reviews, which are often
humorous, descriptive, and helpful.
Leafly also modestly covers other
cannabis topics.
Leafly.com

Marijuana Policy Project

MPP is the largest organization in the U.S. dedicated to ending marijuana prohibition. Their focus is on championing states' rights, as well as regulating marijuana like alcohol. If you want to find out or get involved in the legalization battle, visit MPP's site. *mpp.org*

National Hemp Association

This non-profit Web site advocates for the growth and development of the hemp industry. They primarily serve farmers, processors and manufacturers, researchers, and investors. If you want to learn about or support the use of hemp, this is a good place to start. *NationalHempAssociation.org*

NORML

NORML is a strong site to start with if you are just getting acquainted with marijuana, have health questions, or want to help legalize marijuana. As stated on their Web site, "NORML's mission is to move public opinion sufficiently to legalize the responsible use of marijuana by adults, and to serve as an advocate for consumers to assure they have access to high quality marijuana that is safe, convenient and affordable." Their information on state issues is especially helpful and specific. *Norml.org*

Project CBD

This non-profit association, which has been around since 2010, promotes and publicizes research into the medical uses of CBD and other parts of the cannabis plant. They provide education for doctors and health workers (via seminars), and educate patients, industry professionals, and the general public. Part of their mission is to help physicians and researchers collect data to determine the effectiveness or lack of effectiveness of CBD as medicine and to review CBD-rich strains and products. *ProjectCBD.org*

The Cannabist

The Cannabist is one of the leading journalistic sources on the marijuana industry. Based in Denver, CO as part of the *Denver Post,* it was launched by journalist Ricardo Baca. Cannabis chef Laurie Wolf and other experts contribute. The Cannabist was the first site supported by a major newspaper and dedicated editor. *Cannabist.co*

Wake and Bake

The wakeandbake.co Web site focuses on cooking with cannabis. It is full of humor, great tips gained from Corinne Tobias' years of experience in the kitchen, and recipes. The site includes product reviews, a very good dosing calculator, and personal, engaging stories. *Wakeandbake.co*

WORKS CITED

"2014 Farm Bill - Sec. 7606." Sec. 7606 of the 2014 Farm Bill - Legitimacy of Industrial Hemp Research, www.votehemp.com/2014_farm_bill_section_7606.html.

Americans for Safe Access 2018. *Medical Marijuana Access in the United States.*

BDS Analytics and New Frontier Data. 2017. "The CBD Report." *Hemp Business Journal*

Boire, Richard Glen, and Feeney, Kevin. 2007. *Medical Marijuana Law.* Ronin.

Booth, Martin. 2005. *Cannabis: A History.* Picador.

Brown, David J. 2011. "The New Science of Cannabinoid-Based Medicine: An Interview with Dr. Raphael Mechoulam." *Mavericks of the Mind.* mavericksofthemind.com/dr-raphael-mechoulam.

Carbonnel, Katrina Vanderlip. 1980. "A Study of French Painting Canvases." *Conservation OnLine.* cool.conservation-us.org/jaic/articles/jaic20-01-001.html.

DEA (Drug Enforcement Administration). "A Tradition of Excellence: A History of the DEA." DEA Museum & Visitors Center - Museum Exhibits. www.deamuseum.org/deahistory-book.

———. "Drugs of Abuse - Marijuana." www.dea.gov/pr/multimedia-library/publications/drug_of_abuse.pdf#page=74.

———. "Drug Scheduling." DEA / Drug Scheduling. www.dea.gov/druginfo/ds.shtml.

Fernández-Ruiz, Javier, et al. "Cannabidiol for neurodegenerative disorders: important new clinical applications for this phytocannabinoid?" *British Journal of Clinical Pharmacology* 2013 Feb;75(2):323-33. doi: 10.1111/j.1365-2125.2012.04341.x.

Frontline. 1998. "Busted: America's War on Marijuana." PBS. www.pbs.org/wgbh/pages/frontline/shows/dope.

Gabriel, Barbara. 2018. "Most Older Americans Support Medical Marijuana." AARP. www.aarp.org/health/drugs-supplements/info-2018/medical-marijuana-pain-prescription-fd.html

Gallup, Inc. 2016. "One in Eight U.S. Adults Say They Smoke Marijuana." news.gallup.com/poll/194195/adults-say-smoke-marijuana.aspx.

Ganesan K, and Xu, B. "Molecular targets of vitexin and isovitexin in cancer therapy: a critical review." *Annals of the New York Academy of Sciences* 2017 Aug 1401(1):102-113. doi: 10.1111/nyas.13446.

Gorman, Sean. 2014. "Webb Says U.S. Has 5 Percent of World's Population, 25 Percent of Its 'Known' Prisoners." Politifact. www.politifact.com/virginia/statements/2014/dec/15/jim-webb/webb-says-us-has-5-percent-worlds-population-25-pe.

Gupta, Sanjay. 2013. "Dr. Sanjay Gupta: Why I Changed My Mind on Weed." CNN. www.cnn.com/2013/08/08/health/gupta-changed-mind-marijuana/index.html.

Hillin, Taryn. 2015. "Science Says Twenty-Somethings Probably Shouldn't Smoke Weed." *Splinter*.

Hindocha, C., Freeman, T.P., Winstock, A.R., Lynskey, M.T. 2016. "Vaping cannabis (marijuana) has the potential to reduce tobacco smoking in cannabis users." *Addiction*. 111(2):375. doi: 10.1111/add.13190.

Kalata, Jean. 2004. "Medical Uses of Marijuana Opinions of U.S. Residents 45+." *AARP the Magazine*. assets.aarp.org/rgcenter/post-import/medical_marijuana.pdf.

Klein, Zack. 2015. *The Scientist: Are We Missing Something?*

Mack, Alison, and Joy, Janet E. 2001. *Marijuana as Medicine?: The Science beyond the Controversy*. Washington D.C., National Academy Press.

Manniche, Lise. 2006. *An Ancient Egyptian Herbal*. British Museum.

Marist Poll. 2017. *Weed & the American Family*. maristpoll.marist.edu/yahoo-newsmarist-poll

Mechoulam, Raphael. "The Story of Raphael Mechoulam and the Endocannabinoid System." *The Scientist*. mechoulamthescientist.com.

National Commission on Marihuana and Drug Abuse 1972. "The Report of the National Commission on Marihuana and Drug Abuse." *Marihuana, A Signal of Misunderstanding*. Schaffer Library of Drug Policy. www.druglibrary.org/schaffer/Library/studies/nc/ncmenu.htm.

Pacher, Pál, and Kunos, George. 2013. "Modulating the Endocannabinoid System in Human Health and Disease - Successes and Failures." *FEBS Journal* vol. 280, no. 9: 1918–1943. doi:10.1111/febs.12260.

"Painting Surfaces." *Oil Painting Art - Painting Surfaces*. art-handbook.com/surfaces.html.

Pellechia, Thomas. 2018. "Alcohol Sales Dropped 15% in States with Medical Marijuana Laws." *Forbes*.

Perlmutter, Ed. 2017. "Perlmutter Bill Would Give Marijuana Ventures Access to Banking System." perlmutter.house.gov/news/documentsingle.aspx?DocumentID=1717.

Seppa, Nathan. 2010. "Not Just a High." *Science News* vol. 177, no. 13: 16–20. JSTOR, www.jstor.org/stable/25677928.

Szalay, Jessie. 2015. "What Are Flavonoids?" LiveScience. www.livescience.com/52524-flavonoids.html.

Watts, Geoff. 2006. "Cannabis Confusions." *British Medical Journal*. BMJ Publishing Group Ltd. www.ncbi.nlm.nih.gov/pmc/articles/PMC1336775/.

Wing, Nick. 2016. "Police Arrested Someone for Marijuana Possession Every 51 Seconds in 2014." *The Huffington Post*. www.huffingtonpost.com/entry/marijuana-arrests-2014_us_560978a7e4b0768126fe6506.

Wolf, Laurie. 2013. "How to Make Cannabutter in 7 Steps." The Cannabist. www.thecannabist.co/2013/12/27/kitchenweed/1244.

ABOUT THE AUTHOR

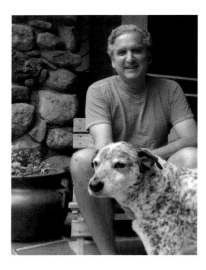

Born in Denver as one of 13 children, Rob Mejia grew up like most kids—playing sports, hanging out with buddies, and smoking a little weed. A talent for tennis (and strong academics) led Rob to Georgetown University. After a decade or so in NYC publishing, Mejia discovered his real business passion: licensing.

When his beloved sister Theresa passed from cancer, he questioned why none of her many doctors had suggested cannabis as a source of relief from her years in agonizing pain. Thus began his journey to learn more.

Through academic and ethnographic research over the course of five years, Rob collected the stories of the community and the questions of his friends. The result was Our Community Harvest, a company focused on cannabis knowledge. OCH offers courses, seminars, and cooking instruction for the curious.

Rob is the proud father of six sons and partner to his equally enthusiastic wife, Beth. He loves to play tennis, make deep-dish pizzas, and now and then, smoke a little weed.

PHOTO CREDITS

Photography credits are listed by page; all starred credits are courtesy the listed name via istockphoto.com.

cover, 8, and throughout, shutterstock.com/Bokasana; 11, Beth Ann Mejia; 16, Barney Warf; 17, Sonia Bonet*; 18, powerofforever*; 22, ctrlaplus1*; 25, Smart*; 26, sbostock*; 30, Mark Coffin; 31, NataGolubnycha*; 32, elenabs*; 33, AlenaPaulus*; 38, elenabs*; 39, Bacsica*; 46, elenabs*; 47, Rouzes*; 47, Yarygin*; 49, RylandZweifel*; 49, CaraMaria*; 50, nathanphoto*; 51, bondgrunge*; 53, Ben-Schonewille*; 56, thegoodphoto*; 60, SageElyse*; 62, Nastasic*; 66, smontgom65*; 67, OlegMalyshev*; 67, UrosPoteko*; 78, bert_phantana*; 78, Nastasic*; 80, Dmitry_Tishchenko*; 84, AHPhotoswpg*; 87, rgbspace*; 89, RapidEye*; 97, JulNichols*; 99, tCheck; 101, Ardent Cannabis; 102, LEVO; 102, Corinne Tobias; 110, geemly*; 112, boblin*; 114, thesomegirl*; 117, Roxiller*; 120, vikif*; 126, Creative-Family*; 127, Lisovskaya*; 128, FreezeFrameStudio*; 132, Chepko*; 134, jenifoto*; 135, zefirchik06*; 138, cveltri*; 139, DebbiSmirnoff*; 143, jacoblund*; 144, haoliang*; 146, robynmac*; 150, Emily Blanchfield; 158, Tim Shu; 176, Renae Knorr (@renaelareephotography). Rob Mejia, 11, 24, 62, 74, 83, 150.

MEASUREMENT CONVERSION CHART

¼ ounce	7 grams
½ ounce	14 grams
¾ ounce	21 grams
1 ounce	28 grams
1 pound	500 grams (1/2 kilogram)
2.2 pounds	1 kilogram
Dash or pinch	about ⅛ teaspoon or less
1 teaspoon	5 milliliters (ml)
3 teaspoons	1 tablespoon
1 tablespoon	15 milliliters (ml)
2 tablespoons	1 fluid ounce
4 tablespoons	¼ cup or 2 fluid ounces
16 tablespoons	1 cup or 8 fluid ounces
1 cup	¼ liter
2 cups	1 pint
2 pints	1 quart
1 quart	scant liter
4 quarts	1 gallon

In order to convert Fahrenheit temperature into Celsius (an older name
for Celsius is Centigrade) use the following formula:
Subtract 32, multiply by 5, and then divide by 9

For example, let's convert 200° Fahrenheit into Celsius:
200 -32 = 168; 168 x 5 = 840; 840 · 9 = 93.3 degrees Centigrade

To convert Celsius (sometimes referred to as Centigrade) into Fahrenheit, use the following formula:
Multiply by 9, divide by 5, and then add 32

For example, let's convert 150° Celsius to Fahrenheit:
150 x 9 = 1350; 1350 · 5 = 270; 270 + 32 = 302 degrees Fahrenheit

CANNABIS JOURNAL

This information will remind you what you liked or disliked about particular strains and products. Because we each have a different physical makeup, what works for you may not work well for someone else. If you are diligent about filling out the forms, you'll definitely benefit in the future! For more information on journaling, see page 75.

Name of strain:

Quantity purchased: Date: Price:

Description of product:

Where product was purchased:

Potency (THC vs. CBD) per serving:

Serving size/Amount consumed:

How product was consumed:

Reason for trying this product:

OBSERVED EFFECTS (CHECK ALL THAT APPLY)

- ❏ Euphoria
- ❏ Lack of energy
- ❏ Different levels of pain relief
- ❏ Hunger
- ❏ Increased anxiety

- ❏ Increased creativity
- ❏ Increased focus
- ❏ A feeling of body relaxation
- ❏ Dry mouth
- ❏ Paranoia

- ❏ Extra energy
- ❏ Lack of focus
- ❏ A feeling of mind relaxation
- ❏ Reduced anxiety
- ❏ Sleepiness

- ❏ Other (Write out below)

Describe the initial feelings and effects felt:

Describe the feelings and effects felt at peak:

Describe the lingering feelings and effects felt:

Summary of findings:

RATING:

CANNABIS JOURNAL

Name of strain:

Quantity purchased: Date: Price:

Description of product:

Where product was purchased:

Potency (THC vs. CBD) per serving:

Serving size/Amount consumed:

How product was consumed:

Reason for trying this product:

OBSERVED EFFECTS (CHECK ALL THAT APPLY)

- ❏ Euphoria
- ❏ Lack of energy
- ❏ Different levels of pain relief
- ❏ Hunger
- ❏ Increased anxiety

- ❏ Increased creativity
- ❏ Increased focus
- ❏ A feeling of body relaxation
- ❏ Dry mouth
- ❏ Paranoia

- ❏ Extra energy
- ❏ Lack of focus
- ❏ A feeling of mind relaxation
- ❏ Reduced anxiety
- ❏ Sleepiness

- ❏ Other (Write out below)

Describe the initial feelings and effects felt:

Describe the feelings and effects felt at peak:

Describe the lingering feelings and effects felt:

Summary of findings:

RATING:

INDEX

MORE GREAT BOOKS *from*
SPRING HOUSE PRESS

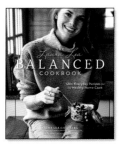

**The Laura Lea Balanced
Cookbook**
978-1940611-56-3
$35.00 | 368 Pages

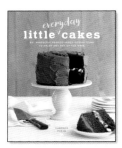

Little Everyday Cakes
978-1940611-67-9
$22.95 | 160 Pages

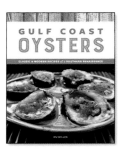

Gulf Coast Oysters
978-1940611-76-1
$24.95 | 216 Pages

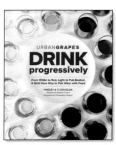

Drink Progressively
978-1940611-58-7
$27.00 | 240 Pages

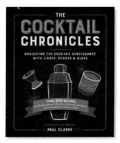

The Cocktail Chronicles
978-1940611-17-4
$24.95 | 200 Pages

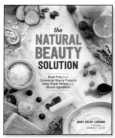

The Natural Beauty Solution
978-1940611-18-1
$19.95 | 128 Pages

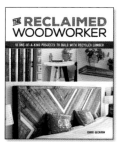

The Reclaimed Woodworker
978-1940611-45-9
$24.95 | 160 Pages

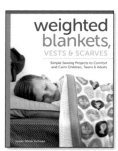

Weighted Blankets
978-1940611-46-4
$12.99 | 48 Pages

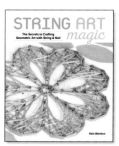

String Art Magic
978-1940611-73-0
$22.95 | 144 Pages

SPRING HOUSE PRESS